Lilias, Yoga, and Your Life

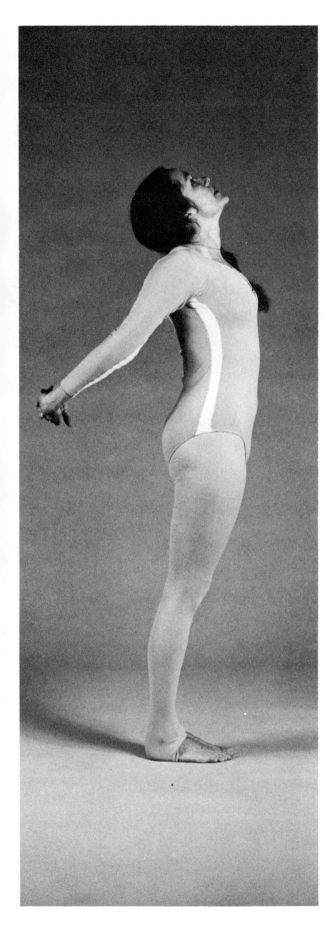

Lilias, Yoga, AND Your Life

Lilias M. Folan

Collier Books
A Division of Macmillan Publishing Co., Inc.
New York

I would like to dedicate this book to my dear teacher and inspiration, H. H. Swami Chidananda and to his teacher, Holy Master Sivananda, the founder of the Divine Life Society, Rishikesh, India.

I offer this work up to the Light of Lights with thanks, gratitude, and love.

Copyright © 1981 by Lilias M. Folan

All rights reserved. No part of this book may be reproduced or transmitted in any form or by any means, electronic or mechanical, including photocopying, recording or by any information storage and retrieval system, without permission in writing from the Publisher.

Macmillan Publishing Co., Inc.
866 Third Avenue, New York, N.Y.   10022
Collier Macmillan Canada, Inc.

Library of Congress Cataloging in Publication Data
Folan, Lilias M
   Lilias, yoga, and your life.
   Bibliography: p.
   1. Yoga, Hatha. I. Title.
RA781.7.F64   613.7'046   80–22579
ISBN 0–02–080060–6

First Collier Books edition 1981
8   7   6   5   4   3
Printed in the United States of America

DESIGNED BY RON FARBER

All photographs in this book were taken by **Gordon Baer** of Cincinnati, Ohio, with the exception of the photos of Bonita Bradley (*Yoga Journal*), Craig Virgin (John Esser), Buhler, Oates, and Trabert (Jim Schneider), and Noel Tyl (Sandy Underwood).

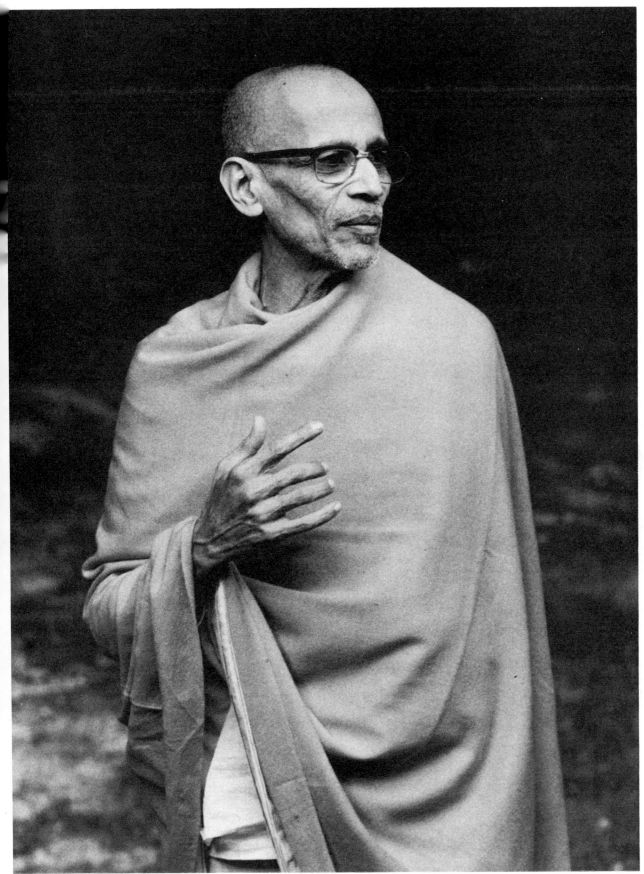

Sri Swami Chidananda

Contents

Preface

The Namaste gesture is an ancient greeting from India. It is a very special way of acknowledging a friendship. The palm of one hand is pressed against the other, meaning: "I greet and acknowledge that the spirit and light within you are the spirit and light within me. We are one."

And so to you, my unseen class, I raise my hands and say Namaste. It is you I salute. It is for you that I write this book.

We are all part of a Scattered Brotherhood: men and women walking on many paths, yet all climbing the same mountain and gazing upward toward the highest goals.

The peaks of self-knowledge are dimly etched in the far-distant mountain mist. At times it is easy to become discouraged. The way can be silent and lonely. The path narrows. The breath becomes short; the feet weary. Yet, as you rest upon the large boulders along the way, give yourself a chance to look back. Ponder how far you've really come! See how the steep climb has offered you creative ways to look at and to know yourself, and how it has given you numerous opportunities to grow. This fresh perspective will help you to realize that although you aspire to reach the summit, experience is interesting, *the journey is the key*!

What are these mountain peaks we hope to attain? For each man and woman the goals vary. They change from year to year as our inner vision expands its capacity for growth and understanding. For some, the summit is the perfection of a Hatha Yoga posture; for others, a more joyful, balanced day—no matter what that day may bring. And for others, the mountaintop is a deeper understanding of answers to important personal questions such as, "Who am I?" "Where am I going?" "Why am I here on earth?"

Many of you have written to me sharing your deepest feelings about yourselves, your families, the ups and downs of living, and your own growth process. You've shared with me the changes that Yoga has brought to your lives, how it has helped to strengthen you physically and mentally, and how it has affected your spiritual outlook on life.

It is very interesting to me to see how your questions have changed over the years. Now there are fewer questions on "how to firm the stomach" and more related to "how do I get my own act together?" It's really been quite exciting!

I am so grateful that you have shared yourselves with me. As I look around and see your progress and growth, I realize that your triumphs are my triumphs; your discomforts, my discomforts. We are not meant to make this long mountain journey alone. The members of our Scattered Brotherhood need to support one another with compassion and love.

It is difficult to imagine anything changing the ancient form of physical culture called Hatha Yoga. But, believe me, it is happening today through a synthesizing process. We are learning how to enrich our lives by combining aspects of *all* available methods and approaches. As a result the ancient Hatha Yoga techniques now vibrate with new energy.

The art of teaching the technical aspects of Hatha Yoga exercises has also changed in a significant way. Teachers from all over the world now advocate preconditioning exercises before attempting the Asanas, an approach not found in the old India texts. I do not consider this a watering-down or a departure from the Yogic traditions, but something that will enrich what we have gratefully inherited from the East.

The purpose of this book is to share the many ways that Hatha Yoga can contribute to your way of life—not as something "way out" or "peculiar" but something real and eminently usable whatever your lifestyle or occupation.

I've tried to include a wide range of exercises, postures, and relaxation and breathing techniques of Hatha Yoga to meet your varying needs. The athlete will be able to use the stretches to ward off possible injuries from jogging, football, hockey, and other sports. The performing artist will learn the secrets of professionals on how to deal with tensions and restore energy. The person with a backache will discover easy postures that will relieve pain and tension in a mere twenty minutes. The business person will find a few tension-relieving, energizing exercises that are simple to do while sitting at a desk. The pregnant mother will learn postures that will prepare her body for delivery and restore her muscle tone and body shape after delivery. Retired men and women will enjoy trying the easy postures and breathing exercises that will help them to stay supple, energetic, and optimistic.

Whatever your lifestyle I will show you how to incorporate Yoga into your daily routine in a creative, realistic, and practical way.

The large rocks and shady trees along the path have offered us a cool rest. It is time to be on our way. As we walk, let us remember not only to look down at the short, limited strides of our feet, but also to raise our eyes. Look up! See the crystal-clear vision that lies just ahead. Take a deep breath and smile. We are on our way to becoming. . . .

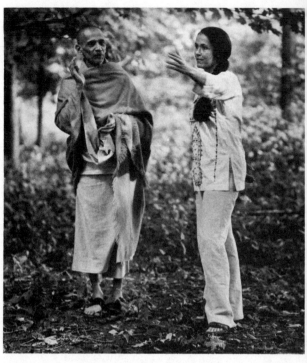

Look Up! See the Crystal Clear Vision That Lies Ahead.

ॐ

Radiant Immortal Soul !

    Blessed Seeker of Health & Happiness,

        Peace be unto you and the Joy of the Divine. To you who are the Reader of this dedicated work "Lilias, Yoga and Your Life" I send you my greetings and this message of my good wishes. May your study of this book be rewarding and beneficial to you in terms of better health, enhanced energy, better understanding of yourself and others and inner Peace and the Joy of a deeper awareness of your real and essential Being.

        Lilias is a sincere teacher and a friend-in-deed. She wishes to share with you what she has found gainful and enriching to her in her own life. She is a bridge between the ancient & the modern, the mystical and the practical. Her approach to yoga is creative and progressive. She blends the discovery of the Vedic seers with the modern knowledge of our present day savents and presents you with a practical guide to self-unfoldment, poise, peace and inner illumination. God bless you with all these ! I congratulate both her as well as YOU !

Jai Gurudev.

                      Swami Chidananda ॐ

Acknowledgments

Many thanks to Dr. Thomas Todd for his medical advice, to Diana Noyes and Mejeh Eggerding for their support when I needed it, to Minette Hoffheimer and Joy Rolfsen for their valuable help, and to all the Yoga teachers all over the world who have inspired me to reach, stretch, and grow, and especially to B.K.S. Iyengar and Bernard Rishi.

And, finally, my thanks to my family, Bob, Michael, Matthew, Melinda, and Marcia. I love you all.

Lilias, Yoga, and Your Life

I woke up one spring morning a number of years ago with a profoundly disturbing thought: "I have everything. I have a kind and loving husband, two handsome, healthy sons, a white clapboard house, two cars in the garage, a boat on Long Island Sound, and a golden retriever. Yet, I am not happy. Why?" Soon many questions began pushing me to seek some other answers to the *whys* of life.

Spiritual teachers of the past and present say that when we have the eyes to see, we will see; when we have the ears to hear, we will hear. The eyes and ears of which they speak are the inner senses attuned by our inquiring and reaching out in the desire to grow. As soon as I began to question and yearn, the right books, friends, classes and teachers came into my life. I recognized that I needed help in coping with the stresses and strains of my everyday life as a mother and as a woman. I also wanted to uncover my own creativity, uniqueness, and spirit. I sensed that an exercise routine might be a good start.

I decided I had to find a routine I would stick with; one that would challenge me physically and mentally; that could help me with my occasional times of low energy, depression, fears, worries, or negative attitudes; and one that wasn't boring.

I turned to Yoga. Like many other Americans, my first encounter with Americanized Yoga was through Jess Stearn's book *Yoga, Youth and Reincarnation*. It spoke honestly and openly about Yoga students, their questions, and their problems. Very soon I too was able to relate Yoga to much within my own life.

As an inexperienced Yoga student, I had many misconceptions about Yoga, ones that you too may have. At first I thought Yoga was a religion that would require me to abandon my own Christian beliefs. I learned that was not so and that Yoga could provide me with the glasses to clarify and study my own religion. I also learned that Yoga had nothing to do with astrology, psychics, reincarnation, yogurt, or lying on a bed of nails.

My reading revealed that Hatha Yoga and Yoga are two separate but related matters. Imagine Yoga as a tree with four large branches; devotion, or the Yoga of love centered on the Divine, (Bhakti Yoga, which includes Mantra Yoga); philosophical analysis and discrimination or exploration of the intellect (Jnana Yoga); the way of action (Karma Yoga); and the royal way or Yoga of inner concentration (Raja Yoga). Hatha Yoga is a small branch of Raja Yoga.

Those who developed Hatha Yoga in ancient India developed a simple system of eight or ten poses that has evolved into the elaborate techniques of today. I have never felt you *had* to adopt the Hatha

I

Yoga and Your Life

Yoga philosophy to enjoy the improved physical and mental well-being that many people experience with regular practice of the Hatha postures (Asanas), breathing techniques (Pranayama), and concentration exercises (Chandra). Gradually and naturally, most Yoga students find themselves awakening to the higher values in life, and passing through the doorway of Hatha Yoga at higher pathways that lead to new goals.

STARTING HATHA YOGA

Most readers should spend the first week practicing the tension-relieving exercises in chapter 3, "Creative Relaxation." Always read instructions thoroughly before attempting any exercises. Go slowly into "Building Blocks" and "Stepping Stones." Older beginners or those who have not exercised in a long time should start with chapter 16, "Nice and Easy Yoga." Preschoolers should be guided through the routines found in chapter 18, "Hatha Yoga Exercises for Preschool Children." Pregnant women should focus on the chapter addressed to them after consulting with their doctor.

THE GIRLS

By Franklin Folger

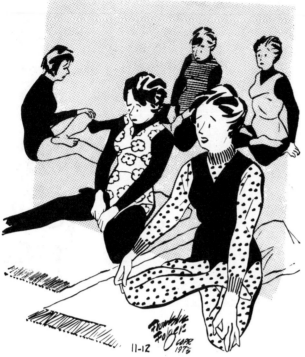

"I'll tell you what I'm meditating on — I'm meditating on how I'm going to get out of this position."

CONTACT LENSES AND GLASSES

Eye doctors feel that it is very safe to wear contact lenses and glasses for many sports, and Hatha Yoga is no exception. However, we sometimes do tension-relieving exercises that require squeezing the eye and facial muscles. Since contacts are likely to pop out, please do the facial squeezes with care and keep your contact-lens case close at hand. Remove contacts and glasses before your deep relaxation.

SPECIAL HEALTH PROBLEMS

Consult your doctor and obtain permission to practice these Hatha Yoga exercises if you have a special problem. This is essential for a student who has undergone major surgery, or suffers from heart trouble, hypertension (high blood pressure) or orthopedic problems. It is recommended that such students consult a Yoga therapist, that is, a Yoga teacher with a medical background such as physiotherapy.

Special notes for women: Questions about practicing during your menstrual cycle, or when pregnant, or when wearing an IUD, and other similar questions are answered in detail in "Yoga During Pregnancy."

TIME OF PRACTICE

The best time to practice is early in the morning, late afternoon, or before bed. Exercising in the morning is not easy for the body because of stiffness, but with practice you'll find that stretches and postures performed in the morning get the circulation going, improve stamina, energize you, and clear the mind. In the evening, the body moves freely, and postures are done with more ease. Evening practice removes the body fatigue and negative tensions of the day, leaving the body and mind refreshed.

Postures should be done on an empty stomach. I try to give myself three hours between a meal and teaching a class. In the morning, I can tolerate a little tea, whole-wheat toast and sometimes, hot cereal before practice. A heavy meal before practice makes most people feel nauseated, headachy, and heavy.

WHERE TO EXERCISE AND WHAT TO WEAR

Avoid exercising in hot sunshine or in drafty, cold rooms. Be sure the floor is covered with thick carpet, or use a good quality mat such as the one shown in this book.

Wear loose-fitting warmups, jogging suits, leotards, or footless tights. Do not try to exercise in blue jeans. They are much too confining. On cold winter days in unheated gyms, layer up with leg warmers, sweaters, or vests, and peel down as you get warm. Wear warm socks, and then remove them for standing postures. Nothing feels worse than being cold during relaxation. Throw a sweater, coat, or blanket over you for deep relaxation.

Do you practice each day whether you want to or not?

Yes, I try to practice each day. The length of time varies according to my schedule.

Exercising alone, day after day, month after month, can sometimes leave me totally uninspired. Sometimes there are days when my body feels so tired and stiff that lying down on my exercise mat feels like a chore. I've found that coping with moments such as these is a part of my growing process. It gives me the opportunity to learn about myself.

Probably one of the most valuable insights came to me at a time when I was going through a lot of inner stubbornness about my own daily practice. I kept observing myself saying, "I'll do it tomorrow," and that tomorrow never came. I was sure that I was the only person in the world who was such a procrastinator. Soon, a good, old-fashioned case of guilt feelings would follow. "You are a teacher! Where is your enthusiasm!"

The solution to my problem came through listening to a wonderful spiritual teacher who has been a great inspiration and light in my life, Swami Chidananda. He helped me to understand that procrastination is just a part of the human condition; everyone has it in one form or another. He told me about a plaque his teacher Master Sivananda had, on which was printed D.I.N.—Do It Now! It was both freeing and comforting to me to understand that procrastination is a weakness common to many human beings. I happily accepted it within myself, and that acceptance allowed me to move forward.

So now a slip of white paper boldly printed with D.I.N. hangs on my refrigerator door and bathroom mirror.

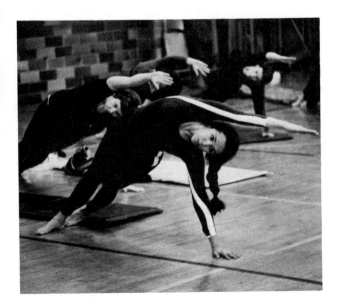

Lilias and Class

2
Questions and Answers

I am a woman, thirty-five years old, with a terrific husband and three children. I started Yoga three months ago, and I love every minute. Basically, I'm a lazy person when it comes to exercising, but I've found Hatha Yoga so fascinating that I've stuck with it. To my surprise, I am really beginning to change. My dress size is down one size; I've lost inches and a few pounds. My entire body feels stronger, looks younger and firmer. My husband appreciates the new me, but feels uneasy that I will change too much. What was your experience, Lilias, when you first started?

All this "change" can seem very threatening to one's spouse. My own marriage went through growing pains as I became increasingly absorbed in Yoga. I am simply not the same person my husband married so many years ago. My husband Bob jokes about the fact that we've been together twenty years, and he has lived with eighteen different women—they've all been me!

As you put more time and energy into your practice, the fruits of your actions will soon become clearer. You will start to notice changes in various ways. Your body will become stronger and more flexible, and you will also find yourself more sensitive and more conscious of your habits.

For example, restaurants with rich foods, smoke, and noise might not be as appealing. As you open up

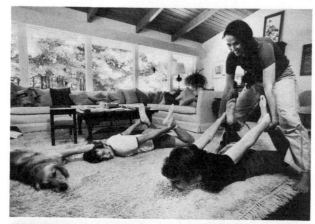

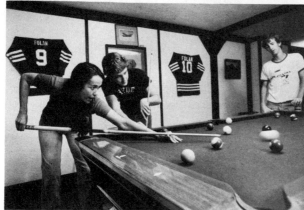

Family Pictures

qualified teacher. Keep in mind that since the needs of each student are different, the characteristics of a good teacher will also vary.

1. Shop around. Go to different classes. Experience different approaches.
2. Notice appearances. A qualified teacher will be clean, neat, and personable, and will exemplify the exercises and philosophy he or she teaches.
3. Check on teaching certification. Although it is not necessary, a teaching certificate indicates that serious time and interest have been invested in the subject.
4. Discuss your search with other friends. Their references can be very helpful when you're considering a new teacher.
5. Listen to your own heart. When all is said and done, therein usually lies the answer.

When is the best time to meditate?

Traditional books of Yoga say that 4:00 A.M. is the best time for meditation. However, my husband would have lasted with me about three days on *that* sort of schedule! It takes compromise. Talk with your family about your need for some uninterrupted time for yourself. Let them express the problems they see with this, and then determine a time for meditation that is best for all of you.

physically, you will open up mentally. The relationships that hide behind masks or revolve around idle chatter may no longer suit you. You will be more open to people and will more probably attract a new group of friends. As you become a more confident, more aware human being, your family and friends will see and instinctively feel the benefits. They may grow as you grow, but the process may not always be easy.

Sometimes I feel nauseated during my practice. It is frightening. Am I doing something wrong?

Possibly you are not breathing correctly with the exercises, or you suffer from vertigo. It also could be a sign of progress because it may indicate that your body is finally confronting your own personality, which is resistant and stubborn. For others, nausea is linked to vertigo and thus arises inner ear malfunction (such as during the Fish). If this is the case for you, omit these postures and movements or try them at another time. Vertigo problems may often get better with time. If this problem persists, consult your personal physician.

How do I choose a Hatha Yoga teacher?

Here are some simple guidelines for choosing a

Occasionally after Yoga classes, I feel depressed— even anxious. This worries me because I thought that doing the exercises would make me feel good.

Many years ago, after an intense Hatha class and deep relaxation, it was not unusual for me to experience occasional feelings of depression. Out of nowhere, waves of sadness washed over my awareness. This experience left me feeling helpless and puzzled. It was doubly lonely because no one else in class out-

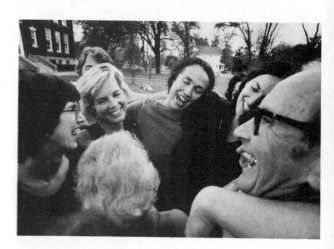

Family Picture

Lilias, Yoga, and Your Life

wardly had this strange reaction to the exercises, relaxation, and positive thinking.

Little is written or explained in the ancient textbooks about students experiencing occasional depression as a direct result of the Yoga postures and breathing. Writing about the subject is easily misunderstood, does not sell books, and does not fill up Yoga classes.

If this happens to you, please, my friend, do not stop Yoga! You are not alone. I think it is a "cleaning-out" process. Yoga gives the muscles and organs a deep massage. Be patient—be grateful. Think of it as some old, dead baggage *that is finally leaving,* not descending upon you!

Daily pressures and the mental stress and strains of life can be wonderously lifted through Hatha exercises, relaxation, breathing, and positive thought. Depressions and sadness, like captive balloons, are finally set free forever! The love of self is then given fresh air and light to grow.

I have heard that people experience great benefits from meditation. How do you meditate?

The benefits of meditation are remarkable. However, when I'm asked "How do I meditate?" I prefer not to answer you too quickly. This is because there are as many ways to meditate as there are people who ask the question. The following steps are meant as a beginning, not an end of your meditation process. As you grow in meditation experience, your "way" will expand also.

I enjoy going through a little preparation before I start my meditation. I light a candle, burn some incense, and set out a lovely fresh flower, or inspirational picture, thus creating a mood *before* I sit down.

Then I set a timer for ten minutes (increase to thirty minutes over a year's time). Put the timer in a drawer so you won't hear it ticking but will hear it ring.

Take your phone off the hook. Tell your friends not to call you at your meditation time.

Sit in a comfortable chair or on a pillow. Do a few neck and shoulder rolls. Take a few deep breaths. Suggest to your body to relax.

Keep a book of inspiration close by; some sort of book that speaks to your heart. (See Bibliography on p. 173.) Read your book for a few minutes to elevate your mind from mundane matters.

Put the book aside and focus your thoughts inward. Close your eyes and ponder those uplifting words. Tune out the outer world and ask yourself, "What did this say to me?" Expand and think about the thoughts of the author. This primes the pump, helping you produce wisdom from within yourself.

Use the Light Prayer (below), or repeat a mantra (a special word or phrase that has meaning and feeling for you) such as, "I am grateful," or, "All is well."

Observe your emotions and thoughts as they are quieted. If your mind wanders, bring it back to your quiet breath or the Light Prayer. Do not wrestle with or get attached to any of your thoughts. Simply watch them as an observer.

If you feel finished with your meditation and the timer has not rung, stay sitting. Pick up your book, but do not walk out. This is important because you are building the habit of meditation. End your meditation with an uplifting thought or a reading that will nurture the mental self and leave you with a feeling of love in your heart.

After your time has elapsed, write down any symbols, random thoughts, or pictures that came to your mind while meditating. Keep what you have written. Your journal will help you to remember the substance of your meditation.

If you feel no results, do not give up! They will come in time. Persevere! Feeling few results is a normal stage in meditation. More rewarding experiences follow.

THE LIGHT PRAYER: SEVEN STEPS TO EFFECTIVE PRAYER

I release all my past, negatives, fears, human relationships, concept of self, my future and human desires to the light.
I am a Light being.
I radiate the Light from my Light centers throughout my being.
I radiate the Light from my Light centers to Everyone.
I radiate the Light from my Light centers to everything.
I am in a bubble of Light and only Light can come to me and only Light can be here.
Thank you God for everything, for everyone, and for me.

James V. Gore
United Research
Black Mountain, North Carolina

Are you a vegetarian?

Vegetarianism has been practiced for thousands of years, and it is often associated with Yoga practitioners. Some of the world's most brilliant thinkers and spiritual leaders have been vegetarians, and some have *not!* One reason I have nearly eliminated red meat, heavy preservatives, and most salt, sugar, and alcohol from my own diet is this: If there is the remotest possibility that I can *prevent* diseases such

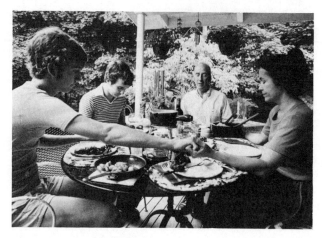

Folan Family Picture

as cancer by adjusting what I put into my body, then why shouldn't I do so?

I remember when I first became conscious of healthier foods and better nutritional habits. My children were young, and I used to feel submerged in hamburgers, ketchup, brownies, and sweetened cold cereals. As the children grew up, their own desire for clear skin, shiny hair, and strong teeth emerged naturally. Their sports activities made them want to find ways of improving their stamina and muscular strength. Their growing interest in health helped the entire family to re-examine our diets and seek ways to improve our eating habits.

The following list summarizes the types of easy dietary changes I found helpful to my own family. I recommend you follow these suggestions to see if you too find they lead you to improved vitality, stamina, digestion, and a better complexion.

Instead of	Why Not Try
White bread	Some of the wonderful 100% stone-ground, wholewheat, rye or cornbreads?
Excess amounts of red meat	Fish and chicken twice a week, an occasional vegetarian dish, using cheese, lentils, soy-beans or garbanzo beans?
White, refined sugars and syrups	Doing without, or sub-stituting honey, dates, pure maple sugar, and syrup?
Cooking oils	Safflower oil, cold pressed oils without propylgallate preser-vative?
Lard, margarine, salted butter	Unsalted butter, nut butter, "Sun Butter" (mix 2 parts butter with one part safflowe oil)?
Mineral salt	No salt at all, sea salt, vegetable-ized salt, so sauce, liquid aminos, miso paste?
Strong condiments, such as mustard, chili pepper, prepared sauces	Vegetable seasonings, onion, celery, garlic, fresh herbs (basil, dill parsley)?
Sugar, sweet desserts, puddings	Fresh fruit, dried fruits?
Vinegar	Lemon juice or pure apple-cider vinegar?
Tea, coffee, "pop," and alcoholic beverages	Fresh fruit and vegetable juices, herb teas, pure water, or lemonade made with honey and mint?
Cold sugared cereals	Granola, whole grains, oatmeal, and wild rice, hot cereal?
Salted nuts	Sunflower seeds, roasted soybeans, pumpkin seeds with sea salt?

I have a terrible time keeping my weight down. Any solutions?

Keeping my weight down while still eating properly takes constant daily awareness. When my weight is up, it definitely affects how I feel about myself, and when my weight is down, I have a difficult time seeing myself as "thinner."

A very big deterrent for me not to "freak out" too often on that hot-fudge sundae is knowing that someone invariably will come up to the table (as I'm hiding behind the whipped cream) and ask, "Are you Lilias Folan?"

Here are a few helpful hints that inspire me to keep on a healthy, happy, and calories-do-count type of maintenance eating diet, which is correct for me and my five-foot-eight-inch, medium-boned frame. I hope these ideas will help you too!

1. A little bit of vanity and value on how you look and feel about yourself is healthy and important! Weigh daily, same time each morning, same clothes, and after you have gone to the bath-

6

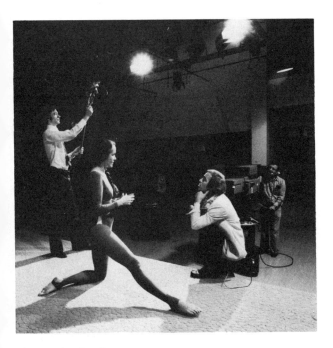

Lilias at the Studio

room. Keep a record of your weight on a nearby chart. Be accurate.

For two weeks, eat nothing made from sugar, or flour, no orange juice, and no whole milk. See if doing this makes a difference in your weight.

2. Try some low-calorie cranberry juice and sparkling water. It tastes delicious, if you are very thirsty in the morning. Keep low-calorie foods, raw vegetables, hard-boiled eggs, cold fish in the refrigerator to eat *before* that sudden, irrational desire to go off the diet hits. Then ask yourself, after you've eaten the low-calorie foods, "Do I still want that other food and why?" Learn to deal with your hunger creatively and respond to your hunger with foods you can have rather than with foods you cannot have.

3. Decrease your attachment and enjoyment of food. Remind yourself that food is tasted on the first three inches of the tongue and that is *all!*

I have been known to place a glazed doughnut, a piece of cake, or some ice cream in my kitchen sink, run water over it, and watch it melt. This is what that goodie looks like in my stomach. Do I still want to eat it? Learn to interpret smells differently, e.g., coffee—indigestion and jitters; fried chicken—greasy; Italian food—heavy and oily.

4. Remember to eat slowly and thoroughly; chew each mouthful about thirty times (boring but better for digestion).

Never eat standing up and try eating occasionally with chopsticks. Put your fork down after each bite.

Try changing your plan of eating. If you eat in front of a TV, go back to the kitchen, or go outside and eat slowly sitting in the sun.

5. Try going on a diet with a friend and join a diet club for two weeks. This can be a help to keep you from slipping away from good diet intentions. But don't consider the whole day ruined if you do slip; just eat less the rest of the day.

6. Try to eat your evening meal before 6:00 P.M. Use children's plates for your main meal and weigh all your food. A kitchen scale is an excellent investment and keeps you honest.

Try not to "think food" during your diet. Stay away from those magazines with photographs of tempting desserts. Avoid dinner invitations for those two weeks. If you must accept, before going drink a cup of hot bouillon or V-8 juice to curb the appetite. Then it will be easier to drink non-alcoholic beverages. Eat the raw vegetable hors d'oeuvres and take small portions of the dinner.

7. Being overweight is treatable. Increased nutritional knowledge, more self-confidence, and new feelings of self-worth are tremendous tools for a healthier, happier, thinner you!

This is a personal question, but do you do anything special to make your hair so thick?

Both my parents had thick, healthy hair. The only thing I do is soak my scalp and hair in avocado oil (available in health-food stores) for twenty-four hours. It washes out beautifully and leaves my hair very shiny!

3

Creative Relaxation— Your First Yoga Lesson

The first lesson to learn is how to relax.

The three steps to relaxation are (1) Focusing and Fixing the Mind, (2) Continuous Suggestion to Relax, and (3) Sensation.

1. *Focusing and Fixing the Mind.* Your inner focus is like a beam of light. Snap on the light. Fix the positioning of the beam on whatever part of the body you wish to relax. Hold it there. Observe. If and when the mind wanders off to other subjects just bring it back, without judgment or frustration, to that part of the body you wish to relax.

2. *Continuous Suggestion to Relax.* After you have focused your attention on that part of the body (e.g., the foot) you wish to relax, give continuous suggestion to the foot to relax deeply. This suggestion to relax is that unseen message being transmitted by the mind to fatigued and tense muscles of the body. In this case, you are doing the suggesting (auto-suggestion, not hypnosis) to each muscle of your body to relax deeply. Even though this continuous suggestion is silent, imagine that every cell of your body hears and is responding to your commands of relaxation.

Take a minute and picture yourself lying in bed repeating the good old American mantra "I am tired" for two hours. How would you then feel? Grumpy? Tired? You bet! Now reverse the idea. Picture yourself saying, "I'm full of energy, joy and balance," for two hours. How would you feel? Of course, uplifted! It is wise to respect the power of your own word and the strength of positive suggestion.

3. *Sensation.* Where you focus your attention, energy follows. After you go through Steps 1 and 2, pause, and feel the sensation of your foot responding. Identify it clearly. Does it feel warm? Cool? Tingly? Pulsating? Heavy? If you feel nothing, this is fine, just go back and repeat Steps 1 and 2. There is no reason to rush; it takes time.

Feeling arises because of the energy you have used to focus upon the muscles you wish to relax. It is the nature of the muscle to feel different when it relaxes totally. It is very much like focusing the sun's rays onto a piece of paper with a magnifying glass. The paper catches fire. So it is with each body part. The energy is caught and focused until the sensation of relaxation arises.

The sensation will be different after each part of the body is relaxed, because *you* are different each day. Sometimes the arms feel long in relaxation and the next day they will feel light or hollow. It is then that you will experience a deep state of relaxation and expanded awareness.

Before you start your relaxation, it would be helpful for you to do a few tension-relieving exercises. They are easy and can be done by anyone regardless of age, size, or previous experience with Yoga. All that's needed is curiosity and a desire to learn. This set of exercises can be done any time and can even be practiced in street clothes.

YAWNS AND STRETCHES

Lie on your back. Bend both knees, feet flat to floor. Place upper arms on floor in a T position. Pushing gently, roll from side to side. This warms up the entire body quickly and feels wonderful.

BACK SCRATCHER

Lie on your back. Bend knees, feet flat to floor. Raise arms over head. Then pretend you are trying to scratch an itch between your shoulder blades, alternating arms.

Press your lower back to the floor and continue with the same side-to-side motion. Then combine the lower-back and shoulder motion stretching arms above head and take a nice big yawn.

Inhale, then exhale, lower arms, straighten knees, legs to floor, and think about your back with your eyes closed. Be aware of how the back muscles feel.

RACK

Lie down, bring arms over your head. Close your eyes and observe the right side of your body, then the left side.

Consciously *relax* the entire left side and stretch the right arm very slowly. Start with the fingers of your right hand, go to palm, wrist, underarm, then to right ribs, waist, hip, outer thigh, knee, calf, foot, and toes. Press lower back into mat. Keep the slow stretching growing and going as if you had a rope on the right wrist and ankle. Take 2 or 3 yawns, bringing air in through the mouth, stretching the skin of the face. Check to see you are *not* tensing any part of the left side as you stretch the right. Hold for about 30 seconds. Release, relax, and observe. Note, with eyes closed, the difference between the right side compared to the left.

Repeat on opposite side.

RULER

Lie on your right side straight as a ruler and arms over head.

Lift your left leg and left arm up 6 inches, parallel to the floor. Left upper arm will be close to left ear; left hand 6 inches away from right hand.

Slowly, slowly, try to lengthen the left side of your body, reaching with fingertips in one direction, and heel and toes in opposite direction. Grow longer on your exhalations, just as if you had a rope on your ankle and wrist. Hold 30 seconds. Then flop onto your back like a rag doll. Lie relaxed for a few moments, just experiencing the freedom of the fall. Observe the body. Let all tension flow out of your fingers and toes.

Turn onto your left side and repeat stretch all the way down the right side of body.

TENSE AND HOLD

Lie on your back, raise arms above the head, with the hands making two separate fists.

Inhale; then, exhaling, lift hips off the mat, pushing heels down to the mat.

Tighten your knees, thighs, buttocks.

Make a "prune face" by contracting your facial muscles, neck, mouth, arms, and hands. Push down between shoulder blades.

Hold from 4 to 10 seconds.

Exhale, release, relax, and observe.

Imagine that the heavy crystals of tension have just been exploded, and that now these small particles are flowing off your ribs and face and out your fingers and toes.

LEMON SQUEEZE

Sit up. Raise arms to T pose. Inhale, stretching both arms out. Lower shoulders from ears.

Exhale, bringing your right shoulder blade in toward your spine. Hold for 3 seconds. Inhale and stretch out again into a T.

Repeat on opposite shoulder.

Now bring *both* shoulders together as you exhale. Hold for 3 seconds. Keep trying to squeeze that lemon between the shoulders.

Inhale, extending both arms, separating shoulders.

Exhale, squeezing both shoulder blades together. Do not raise shoulders.

Release and create a space between shoulder blades by stretching in T, inhaling. Repeat.

Variation

Raise arms in a V. Repeat all the same directions except keep arms in V position.

This exercise is absolutely wonderful for removing that stubborn pocket of tension that lodges between shoulder blades.

THE TANTRUM (POUND YOUR MAT— LET IT ALL OUT)

Lie on your back on the mat. Make arms and legs rigid. Make a good "prune face," squeezing the muscles of mouth and eyes together.

Gently start pounding your mat with your hands as if you are very angry. Keep arms rigid.

Lift heels and bend knees slightly, making the legs loose. Gently start pounding legs up and down the mat.

Keep this movement up for 30 seconds to a minute.

Do not hold sound in. Open your mouth. Let any sound come out freely.

Then stop, relax, and observe the sensations that follow.

I love doing this exercise. It frees locked-in tightness in body, mind, and spirit. Try to let your inhibitions go. Don't worry about feeling silly or self-conscious at the beginning. It is a part of who you are. Think of it as being human.

RELAXATION POSE

Read the following directions completely and slowly 4 or 5 times before lying down for the Relaxation Pose.

Visualize yourself going through all the steps as you read. Your room should be quiet and free of drafts, and your clothes loose and comfortable. Taking a warm shower or sauna before relaxation is especially helpful in preparing your body for relaxation.

Lie on your back, preferably on a mat, or on your bed, under a tree, or on the beach. Close your eyes. Place the feet 20 inches apart (or beyond the width of your hips). Place your arms away from the rib cage, palms turned upward. Pull the shoulders down from your ears and tuck the shoulders blades in toward your spine.

Lift the arms an inch off the ground; let them drop. Lift your upper chest, hips, and legs off the mat separately, then let them flop. Gently press your chin to your chest (keeping back of head to the floor). Release and relax the upper-neck curve of your spine. Inhale, then, exhaling, contact the but-

tocks muscle and press the curve out of your lower back. Release and relax the arch of your spine.

With eyes closed, experience the alignment and balance of your body as you lie quietly on your mat. Now you will alternately identify, tense, and relax, and be aware of each muscle of your body.

First, bring your attention down to your feet. Then, inhale and tense the toes and feet (toes apart if your toes cramp). Hold the breath 3 seconds as you tense the feet. Exhale, relax the muscles of the feet, and observe the sensation that follows. Repeat this process with calves, knees, thighs, entire legs. Then move to the buttocks muscle, sphincter muscle, abdomen, and lower back. Move then to the hands, the entire arm, and into shoulders. For each part of the body, inhale, tense, hold 3 seconds, then release, exhale and observe.

Now move the attention to the face, jaw, area around the eyes, nose and mouth, going through the same procedure. Now relax your entire body by using the three steps to deep relaxation, which is a systematic thought process.

Step 1. FOCUS your attention layer by layer on the skin, muscles, veins, bones, cartilage of each separate part of your body such as your foot.

Step 2. CONCENTRATE continuously on relaxing, say, that foot. (Steps 1 & 2 should take at *least* 15–20 seconds more, if you have the time.) Pause.

Step 3. FEEL THE SENSATION of the foot relaxing.

Please don't rush as you flow from your foot, work to calf, then to the knee, thigh, hip, and then entire leg. Relax abdomen, lower back, upper back, and across chest and shoulders, then down into the hands.

Still going slowly through Steps 1, 2, and 3, bring your awareness to your neck, jaw muscles, tongue, lips, eyes, lines between brows, forehead, behind the ears, top of the head, and finally, relax the scalp.

After going from your toes to the top of your head, go back and repeat the process. Notice that some parts of your body have tensed up again. Relax them again using the 3 steps. The second time will be much easier and the awareness deeper.

With eyes closed, center your attention on the tip of the nose and simply observe the movement of air as it flows through the nostrils. Feel the coolness as it flows in and hits the back of the throat. Then feel and observe the warmth as it flows out. Effortlessly, hold the attention there. If the mind wanders, bring it back to this flow of breath. You will rest both mind and body deeply, in this position. Take anywhere from 5 to 15 minutes to complete the entire process.

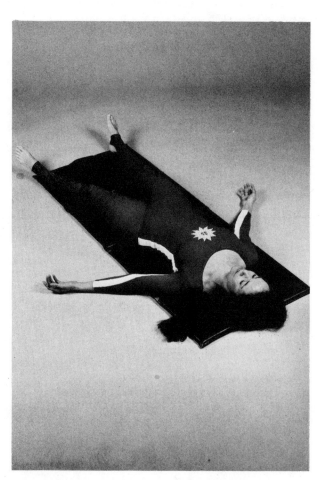

Relaxation Pose

As you come out of relaxation, do so slowly. Before you move, summarize your own experience of relaxation. Then move your feet and toes slowly. Notice how the foot feels. Move your fingertips slowly. Be aware of how each part of your body feels as you begin to move. Deepen your breathing; gently move your head. Deepen your breathing even more. Raise the arms over the head and reach back and yawn, leaving all lethargy on the floor. Ask yourself, "What can I leave on the floor that is old, heavy baggage that I'm not using in my daily life? What can I take home with me into my day, or into my evening?"

Summarize this for yourself. Turn on your left side and, *from your side,* come up into a sitting position. Smile. Give thanks! Feel good about you because you are unique and beautiful. Go into your day taking that which you can use. Feel refreshed, strong, lighter, balanced, ready for whatever awaits you.

Creative Relaxation—Your First Yoga Lesson

4

A Complete Breath

The body can live without solid food for 3 to 4 weeks, 2 days without water, and only 3 to 5 minutes without air. Only when breathing is made extremely difficult do we really appreciate air.

Watch a baby as it sleeps, when breathing is effortless and total—abdomen relaxed, rib cage expanding and contracting with ease. Adults should breathe the same way. But with adulthood comes a certain amount of emotional and physical strain that, over the years, settles deeply into the muscles of the chest, shoulders, throat, and face, thus making breathing shallow and irregular.

So start your day with 10 complete breaths the very first thing in the morning, while still in bed. Take a few deep breaths and do some yawning and stretching.

Visualize with each inhalation how the air nourishes each part of your body and, with each exhalation imagine that all negativeness and tiredness is leaving the body.

Before you try any of the breathing exercises in this chapter, I suggest you read the chapter "Creative Stress—Creative Tension" and that you do the tension-relieving exercises. Tension exercises are quick and easy. It's difficult to breathe properly if one is tight and tense from the day. Rhythmical breathing follows when the body is relaxed.

COSTAL BREATHING

Sit straight, relaxing your shoulders and abdomen.

Close your mouth and breathe through your nose. Wrap your hands around your rib cage (keep your thumb close to your hand), middle fingers lightly touching over diaphragm muscle.

Feel the ribs expanding sideways, almost like an accordion, beneath your hands as you inhale. Look down; watch the space between the middle fingers widen as you inhale, and shorten as you exhale. Make this space even wider as you take 6 slow, even, deep breaths. Continue inhaling to a count of 4 and exhaling to a count of 8. (A count means 1 second.)

Once you feel and see how breathing works, release hands, straighten head and spine, and relax face and jaw muscles.

CLAVICLE BREATHING

We breathe not only up and down, but also sideways. We are all familiar with the front part of our lungs, but little attention is given to the side rib cage and back ribs in our breathing process. The upper areas of the lungs usually remain less active. Clavicle Breathing concentrates more on the breathing that affects the collarbone, the breastbone, and the area between the shoulder blades.

Roll up a washcloth or a pair of socks. Lie down on your mat and place the washcloth or socks between your shoulder blades. Place arms a comfortable distance away from sides. Be aware of the washcloth or pair of socks pressing into your upper spine and skin.

Inhale and, using your imagination, pretend to lift the upper back off the rolled washcloth or socks. Feel the upper chest open and the hollows above the collarbone expand.

Exhale and let your shoulder blades rest or curl around either side of the roll. Still keeping chest open, inhale once again and mentally lift off or roll (shoulders and head stay on floor). Now feel the back of your chest lifting and opening. Observe how the front of the upper chest is also very stretched and expanded.

Exhale, letting your shoulder blades rest (or curl) on either side of the roll.

Repeat this process 5 times. Remove the roll and again repeat the process 5 times. Be *especially* aware of the aliveness of the skin around the area where the roll was placed.

Lilias, Yoga, and Your Life

COMPLETE BREATH

Complete respiration combines the costal and clavicle breathing and integrates them into one flowing, rhythmical movement.

1. Lying on your back, feet and arms comfortably spread apart, exhale the lungs totally.
2. Relax your abdominal muscles. Close your mouth. Open your nostrils wide and back of throat as to stifle a yawn. Now inhale, letting the diaphragm descend, thus allowing the air to be pulled into lungs. The base of the lungs is now filled with air.
3. Expand the ribs, allowing the middle lungs to be filled completely.
4. Continue bringing the air up under the clavicle (the collarbone), the breastbone lifts and even the upper back is expanding.

Slowly exhale to the count of 8, reversing the above process. Starting under the clavicle and working downward to the lower lobes of the lungs, make the air flow in one continuous steady stream. Focus your mind totally on this breathing process.

Helpful Hints

Place a hand towel folded lengthwise in thirds underneath the spine during relaxation. This is extremely restful and keeps the chest gently "open" without strain. It's also helpful for the spine that has become very rounded or rigid with age or disease.

Inhale and exhale through the nose unless otherwise asked.

Try to coordinate breathing and body movements.

The general rule is that when the body is expanded open or stretched, you inhale. When the body is contracted or bent forward, you exhale. When a pose is held, the breathing continues comfortably, rhythmically, and smoothly.

Talk nicely to your body as you inhale deeply into your inner resistance, then let the resistance go on your exhalation.

Breathe in energy, enthusiasm, and newness with each inhalation; exhale tiredness, fatigue, and all negative thoughts.

BHRUMERI BREATH

This exercise will help you to coordinate breathing with body movements and to control long exhalations.

Lie on your back on a mat, arms alongside the body.

Exhale, keeping your arms relaxed alongside your body.

Inhale. With your mouth closed, take a complete breath to the count of 5, raising both arms slowly over your head, fingers toward the ceiling, until the backs of your hands touch the floor.

Exhale to the count of 10, slowly lowering the arms back down alongside your body. Synchronize the motion of your breath with the motion of your arms.

Repeat the above exercise, but on the exhalation, make a "humming" sound like that of a bee (Bhrumeri Breath). Be sure that your fingers touch the floor only after you have exhaled completely. This humming will help you slow down your exhalation.

Repeat the above process 5 times, inhaling quietly to the count of 5, then exhaling totally with the Bhrumeri.

DRAGON BREATH

This breathing exercise is great for quickly pumping oxygen into your system. It gives extra energy and breaks up tense breath patterns. It might make you dizzy at first, but as your system becomes accustomed to this breath, the dizziness should go away. If you still feel light-headed, simply eliminate Dragon Breath.

Standing on the floor, place each thumb on the inside of your hand. Then close the fingers over your thumb. Make your arms very *rigid* through locking the elbows.

Inhale, raising the shoulders up under your ears. Exhale and lower the shoulders.

Repeat the above slowly 5 times. Take a Complete Breath, then 5 more times, and take another Complete Breath.

Repeat the above, each time increasing the tempo. Work up from 5 to 10 shoulder movements.

CLEANSING BREATH

This cleanses the head, quiets the mind and gives energy.

Sit on the mat or in a chair. Inhale completely; then exhale totally through the mouth, making a *ha* sound as you bend forward as far as possible. Then inhale, but this time inhale in little sniffs as you sit up. It will take about 6 or 8 sniffing breaths as you come up to a sitting position. Exhale.

Repeat the above process 3 or 4 times.

A COOLING BREATH

This breath is said to cool the body on a warm day and is helpful in quieting a hungry appetite.

Sit straight.

Curl tongue lengthwise to make a tunnel.

Inhale through the tunnel, pushing the upper lip down to "hold" the tunnel.

Exhale, uncurl the tongue, and press the cooled tongue up against the roof of the mouth.

If you can't curl your tongue, use your fingers to help you. This helps the tongue to get in touch with the muscles needed for the curling action.

The following building blocks are subtle, dynamic principles that are repeated over and over again within the postures. They are not found in traditional Yoga texts. I suggest you read through the instructions and try them out in a relaxed manner each day for a few weeks. Don't feel frustrated if your joints don't move in quite the way you wish. Take your time as you start to combine them with your warmups and beginning Asanas. Reread the building blocks from time to time, but don't struggle with the ideas or concepts. They will all fall into place as you become familiar with the Asanas. Most important, have some fun with them! At this stage of the book, they are like puzzle pieces.

If you are an experienced student of Hatha Yoga, I hope you enjoy this slightly different approach and that it adds awareness and depth to your Yoga practice.

Try all of them in front of a mirror so you can watch your body work.

By understanding and executing the following building blocks, you will (1) develop flexibility and strength in the upper back (thorax and shoulder girdle) and the lower back (pelvic girdle) and (2) see these subtle shoulder and pelvic movements flow throughout many of the postures.

5
Building Blocks

THE THORAX AND SHOULDER GIRDLE

The arms are attached to the body by what is called the shoulder girdle. This girdle is made up of the clavicle (collarbone) and the scapula (shoulder blade). The thorax consists of 12 vertebrae, 12 pairs of ribs, cartilage, and sternum. The sternum is connected to your shoulder girdle with the "glue" of cartilage.

When the thorax and shoulder girdle are well developed and controlled through strength and flexibility, not only will your Yoga postures move freely but also this increased upper-body strength and flexibility will affect your lower body, thus protecting your pelvic girdle from possible injury.

A series of more extensive shoulder girdle and thorax exercises are found in chapters 6 and 7.

SHOULDERS DOWN FROM EARS

Sit or stand in front of a mirror. The arms are straight, as if your hands were holding weights. Elevate your shoulders by raising them up under your ears. Now pull the shoulders down from your ears.

This creates a space between your ear lobes and shoulders. The raised shoulders signal tightness and tension to the muscles of the neck and shoulders. The shoulders are tense and up under the ears. Here shoulders are loose and there is freedom in the neck.

Lie on the mat. Bend your knees, feet flat and 12 inches apart. Tilt your pelvis. Your arms are alongside your body. Palms to mat.

Inhale, rotating the shoulders forward and upward under your ears. Then exhaling, pull the shoulders down from your ears in a smooth, continuous movement. As you press downward, press your shoulders to the floor.

Relax all the muscles of your upper spine. Tension in the muscles of the neck prevents freedom of movement, range of motion, and blood flow to the head area. This move is used in relaxation, standing poses, and the Cobra.

PULLING SHOULDER TOWARD SPINE

Either stand or sit, but with a straight spine.

Straighten your right arm and make a fist with your right hand.

Bend your left arm at the elbow and from behind, grab hold of your upper right arm just above

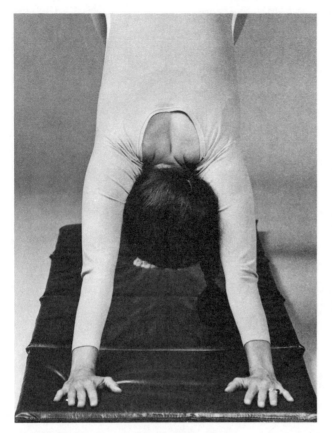

Incorrect Shoulder Pull Down from Ears

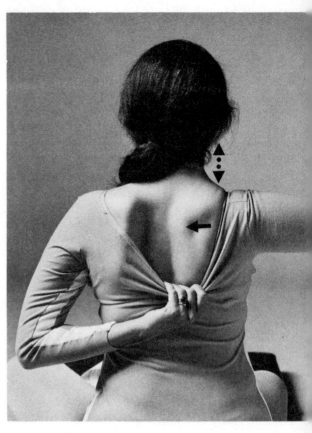

One Shoulder in

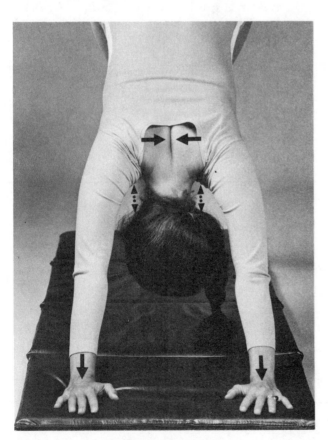

Correct Shoulder Pull Down from Ears

your right elbow. Keep your right elbow straight. Inhale and think tall. Exhale, and pull your right shoulder in toward the center of your spinal column. Look in the mirror to be sure your shoulder is *not up*, but is pulled *down* from your right ear. Hold for the count of 5.

Repeat once more, and then repeat on opposite arm.

This is a simple, yet dynamic action. It is a building block of twists and some one-arm standing side poses.

SQUEEZING BOTH SHOULDER BLADES TOGETHER

Sitting straight in a chair, and again looking at a mirror, place your arms in a T position. I use this phrase often. It means arms directly out, shoulder height, parallel to the floor and palms down. Look into your mirror and pull your shoulders down from your ears.

Inhale; then, exhaling, squeeze both shoulder blades (scapulae) together firmly, like the military posture of squaring your shoulders. Hold to the count of 5.

Lilias, Yoga, and Your Life

Inhale; then exhaling, extend the hands out as far as possible. Feel your arms lengthen. Hold to the count of five. Repeat this extended hold-squeeze-hold-release from 3 to 5 times. You should feel the action in both the front and back of your chest. Remember to create a space between your shoulders.

Variation

Stand up a few feet from the wall. Lean forward and, with your arms straight, place your hands on the wall above your head, feet 2 feet apart, as if you are going to be frisked.

Keep your elbows straight and your head between your upper arms. Open up your fingers like a star. Now walk the heels of your hands downward *only* 12 inches.

Your weight will shift slightly. Hips over heels, bend your knees comfortably. Your weight is now evenly distributed on both feet; relax your toes. No discomfort need be felt on the back of your legs.

Now squeeze both shoulder blades together firmly, applying leverage from the heels of your

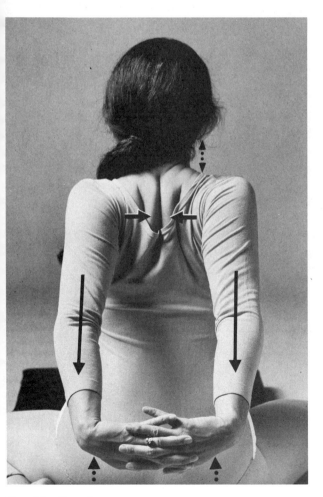

Shoulder Rotation

hands. Feel how the inside of your armpits and the front of your chest open with this shoulder squeeze.

For increased shoulder flexibility, walk the hands down a bit farther.

SHOULDER ROTATION

As you stand or sit on the mat, clasp your hands together behind your back. Inhale and straighten the elbows. Exhaling, pull the shoulder blades together, feel the squeeze between the shoulder blades and notice that your chest also expands.

Inhale again and lift up the sternum. Exhaling, lift the arms a bit higher, still creating a space between the ears and the shoulders. Release and repeat.

This Shoulder Rotation is an especially important building block for the Shoulderstand. (See pages 53–56.)

THE BREASTBONE, OR STERNUM UP

Looking into the mirror, place your hands on your sternum, or breastbone. Lift this area gently upward. Because this sternum is connected to the shoulder girdle, the shoulders will go back easily and the chest will open naturally.

This upward motion may not sound like much, but it is another vital building block for setting into motion the extension or "upness" necessary for backward arches. This building block is used in twists and in standing poses.

LOWER TORSO

PELVIC TILT

Lie down on the mat, bending both knees, feet flat to the mat, and knees and feet 12 inches apart. (Be exact.)

Inhale and arch your lower spine (lumbar curve) gently. Note that in the photo my seat is on the mat, and you can see that my lower spine is arched because I can run my hand beneath the arch. Now you do the same.

Remove your hand. Bring your chin gently to your throat.

Exhaling firmly, contract sphincter, buttocks and abdomen muscles while you flatten and firmly press your lower back to mat.

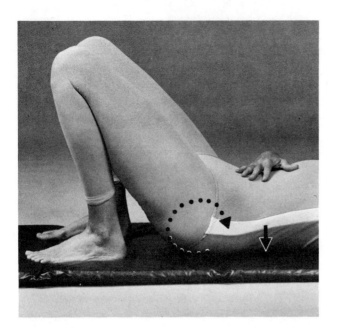

Pelvic Tilt

Inhale. Again *gently* arch the spine and relax the seat and abdomen muscle. Then, exhaling, press the lower spine to the floor, contracting the abdominal, sphincter, and buttocks muscles once again. Hold a few seconds, then repeat 5 times.

Continue with the lower-back-relax-contract action until it becomes easy and fluid. Recheck the angle of your chin. Make sure it is not pointing toward the ceiling in tension, but is pressed comfortably in your throat. This building block is used in the Bridge, Wheel, Sit-back, and standing poses.

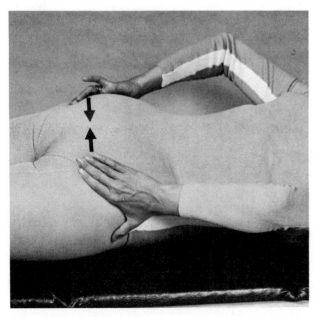

Pelvic Tilt on Tummy

PELVIC TILT ON THE STOMACH

Lie on your abdomen. Inhale, then exhaling, tighten your buttocks muscles and press upper thighs and pubic bone to mat. Repeat three times. This building block is used in the Cobra.

PELVIC TILT WHILE STANDING

Stand up. Tighten the kneecaps and buttocks muscles. The pelvis will tilt automatically. Inhale, then exhale and do the Pelvic-Tilt against a wall.

LENGTHENING THE SPINE

Stand tall.

Take a string and hold one end at your navel, the other end at your breastbone (sternum). Pull the line taut.

Now look down at your chest. Exhaling, make the line between your navel and sternum shorter.

Notice what has happened to the front of your chest. It has collapsed.

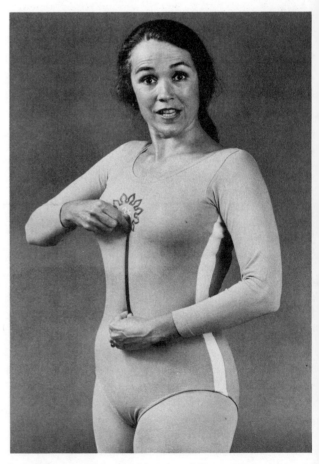

Lengthen Line Between Navel and Sternum

Lilias, Yoga, and Your Life

If you look into the mirror, you will see your spine has rounded.

Inhaling, now lengthen and elongate the line between the navel and sternum. What has happened? The chest is open; the spine is straighter and longer.

Inhale and look at yourself in the mirror. Then exhale and make the line shorter between the navel and sternum. Pause, now inhale and *elongate* your spine by *lengthening* the line between the navel and your breastbone. Note in the mirror what your straightened spine looks like, and *feel* the difference within your body. Remember all poses have not only a front side but also a back side to them. This building block is used in poses such as the Dog and forward bends.

HIP ROTATION AND CONCAVE SPINE

The building-block movements of rotating hips and making the spine concave sound complicated, but are very simple and are part of many different poses. In effect you end up stretching your entire spine from your atlas vertebra (first vertebra beneath your skull) to your tailbone. As you do this, the vertebra of your spine will *descend*, and the muscles of your spine will *ascend*, forming a protective tunnel for the vulnerable spine. When you let your spine fall into a concave position, you are encouraging the natural curvature of your lower back. Yet, take care not to overextend your lower back. Concave does not mean swayback. Please read more about the back in "Back Talk," chapter 13.

In this next exercise, I'd like you to feel with your own hands what this concave hip rotation feels like.

Stand with your seat against the wall, feet 12 inches apart and heels 4 to 8 inches away from the wall for balance. You may bend the knees.

Place your fingers around your hips with thumbs behind the hip bone (the iliac crest). Lean forward, body parallel to the floor. (Your body forms a 90 degree angle). Inhale, then exhale, and now rotate your hips and make your lower spine concave. By this I mean try to bring the perineum (crotch) to the wall.

With your hand, feel the crest of the iliac move beneath the skin. Press those bones downward into the skin of your thighs. Do this a few more times so you really feel this hip-rotation motion.

Now place your hands on your lower back. Relax and slightly round your spine. Feel the little bumps that run in a ridge down your lower back?

Then, exhaling, *rotate the hips and make the spine concave* once more. Feel how the lower-lumbar

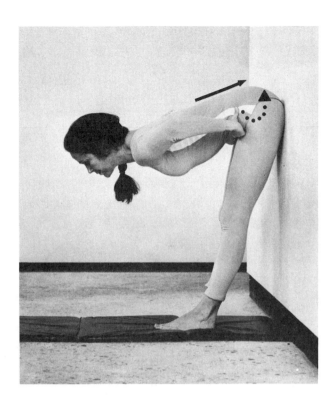

Hip Rotation

back muscles raise up or ascend into action, forming strong ridges of protection, while the vertebrae have descended with the action of the hip. Can you feel the gentle tunnel of the lower back? If not, try the above procedure once more. This building block is often used in forward bends.

STANDING ELONGATION WITH HANDS TO ELBOWS

Try this exercise in your kitchen, using your counter top, or use the top of a bureau, or kneel in front of a chair. The positioning of the arms works the shoulder girdle and tones the abdomen.

Stand (or kneel) a few feet from the counter top. Stretch your arms above your head. Clasp your elbows. Inhale, stretch upward, then exhale, bending at the waist. Lower your trunk to form a 90-degree angle. Place your upper arms on the counter. Squeeze your shoulder blades together.

Adjust your feet so they are beneath your hips. Bend your knees. Rotate your hips downward toward your thighs. Concave your lower back, coccyx bone up to the ceiling.

Release one hand and feel the tunnel of your lower back. Have the little bumps disappeared into your body? If not, return your hands and go through the procedure.

Building Blocks

Inhale, lengthening the line from your navel to sternum. Exhale, pulling your abdomen in and up as you elongate your spine. Inhale, then exhale. Concave your lower back as you rotate your hips.

Inhale and extend the sternum. Exhale as you stretch and open up the buttocks. With a little time this pelvic girdle will become far more flexible.

Helpful Hints

Once you have finished this hand-to-elbow elongation, go through the entire process with arms straight out alongside your ears. Your head stays between your upper arms. Keep your neck free from tension, and remember, no strain. Relax your jaw muscles and your toes!

Also, it is easy to overextend the back of your knees in this pose. Be careful to avoid this condition.

How often have I had Yoga students who worked so hard to develop limberness that they often caused injury to joints and vulnerable areas of the body. Great care should be taken to build strength as well as flexibility in muscles and connective tissue simultaneously.

WARMUPS AND PRECONDITIONING

The Hatha Yoga teachers of ancient times paid very little attention to what we now know as preconditioning, prestretching or warmups *before* executing the Asanas. Perhaps this was because life for the young Indian student was slow and unharried compared to life as we know it today, full of physical, mental, and emotional tensions.

After teaching Yoga for a few years, I began to notice pain and soreness developing within specific areas of my spine where there had been no pain before. My upper neck was constantly sore and stiff after a long Shoulderstand or a quick demonstration of the posture with my body not warmed up. I also noticed a dark, rough brown, callus developing on the skin over the seventh cervical vertebra of my upper neck. My lower back ached and was very painful during and after backbends. A minor sciatic problem that had developed during my pregnancies now flared up painfully.

It was extremely difficult to admit to myself and to others that the pain I was experiencing during the Asanas was caused by one person, me! Obviously, I was doing the Asanas incorrectly. This discomfort compelled me to research my own body in a different way. It forced me to expand my own concepts and techniques of teaching.

The first change I made was to *always* make time for warmups. In this book I refer to these exercises as stepping stones because they pave the way for the poses.

Secondly, I began to analyze each posture as if it were made up of many different building blocks. I discovered that if one part of the posture is weak, the entire structure will be out of balance. Once I had a clearer understanding of the components within each Asana, I was able to work on perfecting their flow and originality.

I strongly urge you to learn from my mistakes. Be sure to warm up and do the conditioning exercises of the postures.

Stepping stones are warmups that pave the way to strong, dynamic, safe postures.

6
Stepping Stones

NECK UP

Lie down on your back and place one of your hands around your throat. Lift your head to look at your toes. You can feel the muscle working beneath your hand. This muscle group is an important factor in the rotation, flexion, and extension of the head. The carotid arteries, jugular vein, and vagus nerve run deeply into these muscles. The front of your neck needs to be as strong as the muscles of the back of the neck and as tension-free as possible. It is a vital stepping stone for the Shoulderstand, Headstand, and other poses.

The first few times you do this exercise you will probably feel a dull muscle ache (not a pain) deep within the muscles of your neck. Do not let this discourage you. Remember, the head is heavy, between 7 and 14 pounds. Therefore, lifting the head up and rotating it from side to side from a lying-down position is not as easy as it looks.

Variation 1
This exercise will firm and tone the skin and lines of the neck. It must be practiced many weeks before starting the Shoulderstand and Headstand. It helps to hold the vertebrae of the upper neck in proper alignment. It is a good warmup for wrestling.

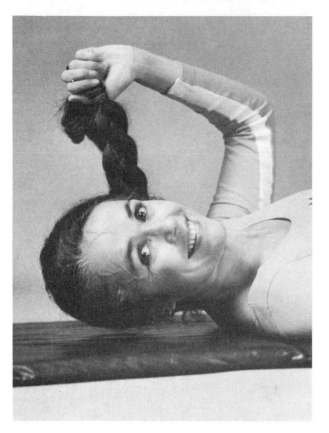

Neck-Up

chin up toward the ceiling. Then slowly bring your chin to your throat. Hold for a few seconds and then return your head to the floor. Always leading with your chin, repeat 4 to 8 times.

NECK TILT

The muscle arrangement of the neck is exceedingly complicated and remarkable. The sternocleidomastoid muscle plays an important part in the rotation, flexion, and even extension of the head.

Knots of tension blocking the energy flow into the head can cause pain, constriction, tension headaches, difficulty in swallowing, facial tension lines, and neck fatigue.

Start by sitting tall or cross-legged in a chair. Both hands are on your knees. Inhale; then exhale and tilt your neck to the left. Do not become the Leaning Tower of Pisa. Your weight should be on your sitting bones (ischium). Your shoulders are in a straight line. Your ear comes down to your left shoulder, but the shoulder does *not* come up to your ear.

After you've gone through this procedure, place your right hand behind your right ear and gently trace the right side of your neck to the tip of your shoulder.

Now continue the downward movement of your right hand and place your fingertips on the floor beside you (or let them hang if doing posture in a chair) but not on your right knee.

Let the weight of your arm pull the neck muscles in one direction and your head pull it in another. Hold the Neck Tilt for about 30 seconds, breathing comfortably.

Slowly release and sit tall once again. Close your eyes and observe the difference in one side of your neck compared to the other. Feel the length of the right side compared to your left.

Repeat the Neck Tilt on the opposite side.

This exercise is especially good for children in grade school gymnastics. The upper neck is especially weak and vulnerable in youngsters.

Lie down on your back with your hands on your thighs, your head on the floor, your face parallel to the ceiling. Lift your head two inches off the floor and look at the ceiling. This is called the start position.

Slowly turn your head to the right, looking over the right shoulder (your right ear is about two inches off the floor); rotate your head back to the start position and hold for 4 seconds. Repeat on the opposite side.

Consciously relaxing your neck and shoulder area, with the back of the head resting on the floor, let your head rock easily from side to side. Add one more rotation by the end of the week, working up to four.

Variation 2

This strengthens the long muscles on the front of the neck and throat.

Place a folded blanket, mat, or gymnastic mat beneath the shoulders. Let your head touch the floor. Roll your chin up toward the ceiling with the head still on the floor. Now, leading with the chin, lift the

LEG RAISES

When the leg raises are done in succession, they will strengthen and tone your pelvic girdle (hip, thigh, and abdominal muscles) and increase your endurance. Moreover, one of the simplest methods of keeping down blood pressure within the veins of the legs is by using the muscles surrounding the veins. Thus, leg raises will help you avoid the problems of varicose veins.

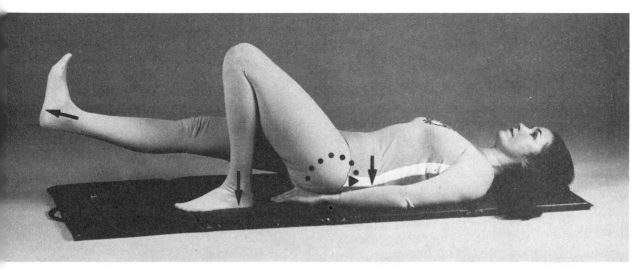

Single Leg Raise

SINGLE LEG RAISES

Keeping the lower spinal curve to the floor is essential during all leg raises. This is done by applying the building block of the Pelvic Tilt and extending your heels throughout the following exercises. In this case, the Pelvic Tilt is used as a "gear" to stabilize the lower back and activate the abdominals.

Because of weak abdominal muscles, you might as a beginner find it difficult to keep the Pelvic Tilt "in gear" throughout the leg raises. If this is so, use your hands as an aid. Place your hands and wrists beneath your seat, thumbs touching. This forms a protective nest for the lumbar curve, and the lower back will stay flat on the floor. Remove your hands as the muscles of the abdomen and lower back become stronger.

Lie on your back and bend both knees. The feet are flat on the floor. Exhale, tilt the pelvis.

Is your spine totally flat to the floor? If not, and the curve is still obvious, straighten your arms; slip the hands beneath your hips, the thumbs touching in the "nest" position. (Note photo.)

Now, raise one leg 8 inches off the mat. Hold this position. Ask yourself, "Am I using all the muscles I can to raise my leg?"

Consciously extend your heel and *contract* your buttocks and thigh muscles, thus using the back and front of your leg.

Without going farther, extend the raised heel and push down on the foot of the opposite leg. This will maintain the steady downward pressure on the lower back that is an absolute *must* for back protection while doing leg raises.

Inhale; then exhale as you slowly lift your leg toward the ceiling to the count of 8. Take another

breath; then exhale as you extend the right heel and slowly lower the leg to the count of 8. The kneecap is pulled up, and the heel is extended. Lower your leg to that point where the curve of the spine starts to strain. Immediately bend your knee and repeat the leg raise 8 times with each leg. Work up to 20.

Helpful Hints

Keep your heels extended and your feet flat during all the leg raises. Do not point the toes.

At first it is not important how many leg raises you can do. What is more important is that you keep the pelvis tilted at all times. Use the front and back of your thighs and buttocks.

After the lower back and abdomen are stronger, then remove your hands from the nest position.

Remember, *no strain on your lower back!*

SINGLE SIDE LEG RAISES

Lie on your back, arms in the T position. Exhale as you raise the right leg and extend the heel to the ceiling. Inhale as you lower the right leg to your left hand, keeping shoulders on the mat. Exhale as you raise the foot up to the ceiling.

Raise the left leg up and lower the left foot to your right hand. Repeat 3 to 6 times with each leg.

SINGLE LEG RAISE WITH TIE

This exercise is especially designed for men and women with great stiffness in the ligaments and tendons of the back of the leg. Work in this way two or three times a week with leg raises, and you'll see

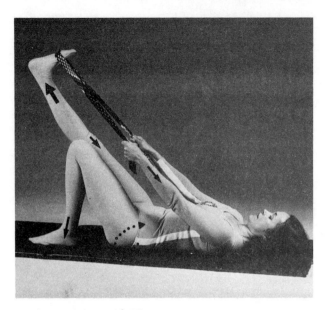

Single Leg Raise with Tie

straighten the legs, and extend the heels to the ceiling.

As you lower the legs, extend the heels, with the pelvis tipped lower to that point where your lower back remains on the floor. The abdomen should be flat.

Just as you are about to lose control, bend your knees. Bring your knees to your chest. Repeat and work up to 10 leg circles with your heels just grazing the mat, making one continuous circle.

Helpful Hints

Remember to place the tie on the ball of your foot, not under the arch.

To eliminate cramping muscles in the front of your legs, stretch the muscles in back of the legs and extend your heels. Keep your upper neck relaxed throughout this movement.

Do not arch or tense your upper neck during the exercise.

LEGS IN V POSITION

These exercises are excellent for firming and strengthening the inner- and outer-thigh muscles. For best results do these every day for six weeks.

Step 1

Lie on your back. Inhale. Exhale. Tilt the pelvis and bend both knees. Lift your legs and extend

results. This is extremely helpful as a warmup for athletes.

Lie down on your back. Bend both your knees. Feet are flat on the floor. Bring your right knee up to your chest. Place a tie or belt around the ball of your right foot.

Straighten your right leg, with heel extended toward the ceiling. Raise the kneecap. Holding firmly on to the tie, bend your elbows up 2 inches off the floor, maintaining the pressure on the ball of your foot. Then, lower your leg until the knees are level to each other. Your arms are now straight, still maintaining pressure on the ball of the foot.

Inhale and extend the heel toward the wall in front of you. Exhaling, contract your abdomen and ribs and tilt the pelvis. Then raise the leg back up toward the ceiling, elbows bent.

Do not move your body. Press the left foot and heel into the floor. This will further tilt the pelvis.

Extend your right heel higher to the ceiling.

Adjust your hand grip on the tie. Elbows should be one inch off the floor. Buttocks stay on the floor. Feel the hip lengthen.

Inhale; then exhaling, lower the leg with the heel *extended* to that point where the knees are level. Then bend your right knee, straighten your leg, and extend the heel toward the ceiling. Repeat the circle 6 times per leg, repeating on opposite leg.

DOUBLE LEG RAISE WITH TIE

Repeat the above procedure. This time place the tie or belt around the balls of both feet as you

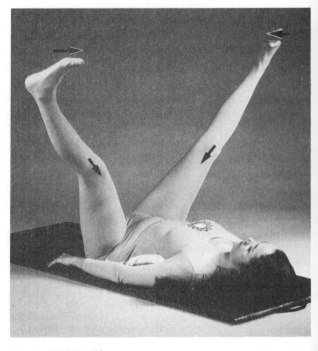

Legs in "V" Position

Lilias, Yoga, and Your Life

heels toward the ceiling; the knees should be straight. Look at your feet and make the big toes touch. The heels should be out as if you were standing pigeon-toed. Keep the heels pushed out during the entire exercise. Keep your hips on the floor.

Step 2

Inhale as you spread the legs apart slowly in a wide V. Exhale, bringing the legs together and crossing your right knee over the left. Repeat this legs apart-together motion 10 times, alternating. Do not hold your breath. Be sure you have a good stretch as your legs go into the V.

Variation

Repeat the body position in the exercise above, but this time place your heels together and toes apart, similar to a Charlie Chaplin stance. Inhale; then exhale, slowly, spreading the legs apart in a V, then legs together, crossing and alternating one knee over the other. Repeat 10 times.

Helpful Hints

Do these V positions slowly. It is easy to overstretch if you bounce your way into these positions.

DOUBLE LEG RAISES

After four weeks of practicing the mechanics of Single Side Leg Raises, you can start Double Leg Raises.

Lying down, bend both knees, heels close to your buttocks, arms straight alongside the body. Bring both knees to your chest as you slide the wrists beneath your buttocks, thumbs touching. This hand position forms a nest for your hips.

Inhale; then exhaling, raise both feet toward the ceiling, heels extended, kneecaps pulled up.

Inhale; then, exhaling, slowly lower both legs to that point where your spine starts to come off the mat. Go back ¼ inch so your spine is on the mat. Hold. Lift the sternum, press your shoulders to the mat.

As you contract the abdomen, exhale, tilt the pelvis firmly, and extend the heels. Check to see if your chin is toward your throat. Hold this position for ten seconds.

Then inhale; then, exhaling, raise both legs slowly up to the ceiling to the count of 8. Repeat 8 times, working up to 15.

Remove your hands from under your seat muscles when you can keep the Pelvic Tilt in gear strongly throughout the entire exercise.

Variation

A variation on this is to lower the legs halfway to the floor. Then extend legs in a V hold. Hold a firm Pelvic Tilt. Inhale, then exhale, and bring the legs together. Repeat three times and work up to five.

DOUBLE LEG RAISES WITH ARMS IN A T

Place arms in a T position.

Bend both knees. Bring both knees to the chest. Flatten your feet; straighten both legs, extending the heels. Inhale and slowly bring both feet to your right hand. Exhale and slowly raise legs up toward the ceiling. Repeat on the opposite side 3 times for each side.

Repeat the above, but this time hold the right ankle to the floor with the right hand. Inhale and slowly raise just the left leg up into a V, then exhale and lower. Repeat 3 times for each side.

Helpful Hints

Keep both shoulders on the mat at all times.

Try to keep both ankles together at all times.

Do the movement slowly. Take 5 seconds, counting *om*-1, *om*-2, *om*-3, etc.

PENDULUM LEG SWING

This is another leg conditioner for strengthening the hip, abdomen, and lower-back area. It will slim the waist, reduce hips and thighs, and tone the abdomen.

Lie down on your back. Your arms should be out to your side in a T position. Look down at your arms, check to see they are shoulder level. The palms are down.

Bend both knees, feet flat on the floor. Tilt the pelvis. Slide your heels down to that point just before your lower back comes off the ground.

Apply pressure to your heels into the floor.

Inhale as you raise the right foot up, heel extended toward the ceiling. Tighten the kneecaps. The buttocks stay on the floor.

Then exhale, as you lower the right leg out to the side, below your right hand, keeping the leg as straight as possible.

If you can reach your wrists without straining, do so.

Take 2 deep breaths. Inhale, then exhale as you lift the foot up to the ceiling. Extend your heel.

Take another breath. On exhalation, bring your right foot down to the left hand. (If you cannot

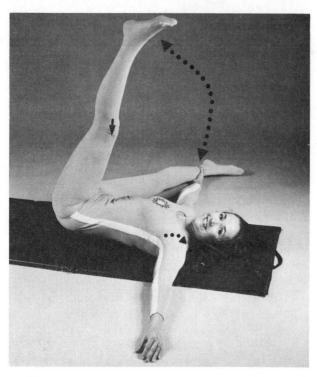

Double Leg Raises, Arms in "T"

reach your wrist, move over a little to the left with your right heel.)

Inhale. On the exhalation, raise the right leg up toward the ceiling.

Inhale; then exhale and lower your leg to the mat.

Relax; then repeat the instructions on the opposite side of your body, 3 to 6 times per leg.

Helpful Hints

Keep your shoulders down throughout the exercise.

Remind yourself that breath and leg movement flow together.

WINDMILL

The Windmill is many of the leg raises rolled into one. It strengthens and stretches the hips and legs, paving the way to standing poses. The abdominal and lower-back muscles and thighs are also firmed and toned.

Lie on your back, arms alongside the body. Bend both knees. Feet are flat on the floor. Knees are hip-distance apart.

Step 1. Bend your right knee to your chest. Inhale.

Step 2. Exhale, and extend your right leg up to ceiling; raise the kneecap up. Extend the right heel.

Step 3. Lower your right leg to 4 inches from the floor, exhaling. Tilt the pelvis. Hold.

Now combine Steps 1, 2, and 3 into one smooth windmill-like motion. Do a round of 10; then rest. Add another 10. In a few weeks, do 20 together. Breathe comfortably.

Repeat on the opposite leg, the 10 plus 10.

For more advanced work, try the Double Leg Windmill, repeating the above exercise with both legs.

Helpful Hints

Press down with foot that is on the mat and use the mat foot as leverage.

Try the nest position of hands when first trying the double leg windmill.

Stop and remind yourself to use both the front and back of the thigh and buttocks muscles as you raise and lower your legs.

Remind yourself that although the Windmill looks like a calisthenic exercise, you are to do it Yogically, with awareness, the proper breathing, relaxing other parts of the body not needed for the actual movement, *and* relaxing after the exercise is complete.

DOUBLE HEEL DESCENT

This intermediate leg raise is done *only* after all leg raises have been mastered and principles understood. An excellent strengthener for the entire back and abdomen. Increases stamina and all-over body strength.

Technique 1

Lie on the mat. Bring arms over the head to touch the floor. Draw your knees to your chest and flatten your feet. Then straighten the legs, extending the heels.

Inhale deeply, then exhale as you lower the legs to that point where your lower back comes off the mat.

Now extend your heels, consciously relaxing your shoulders and neck and facial muscles. Tilt your pelvis with determination! Bring your chin gently toward your chest.

Your entire spinal column should be flat to the floor as you hold for 30 seconds. Relax your face and hands.

Inhale; then exhale, bringing both legs up toward the ceiling. You should be able to do the above without strain before you go to Technique 2.

Repeat three times.

Lilias, Yoga, and Your Life

Bring your knees to your chest then take a few deep breaths and relax.

Technique 2

Extend your heels toward the ceiling. Inhale; then exhale.

Lower your legs *to that point where your vertebrae* start to come off the mat. Then hold for thirty seconds. Tilt yourself to extend your heels and keep the pelvis tilted.

Do not hold your breath. Inhale; then exhale again, lifting your heels toward the ceiling. Repeat and work up to three times.

MALTESE CROSS

This is not an exercise for the beginner. Only when you can do the Double Heel Descent should you start the Maltese Cross.

This tough abdominal exercise is very wonderful as a challenge for the student who has been working with stepping stones and postures for a few months. It can be made more challenging for the advanced student by slowing the count from 10 to 20 for each side. I always feel so virtuous when I've completed the whole circle in both directions—twice! Slowly practice it once or twice a week.

Step 1

Lie on your mat, arms in a T position, legs together.

Inhale; then exhale, tilt the pelvis smoothly.

Bend both knees to the chest and then straighten legs, heels extended and up toward the ceiling.

Step 2

Inhale; then, exhaling, slowly lower both legs to the count of 10, down to 4 inches above the mat. Hold for 5 seconds. The heels should be extended. Breathe shallowly. The body forms a Maltese Cross.

Step 3

Inhale as you sweep the legs in a half circle to the right, 4 inches above the floor, up to the right hand, then above the right shoulder and your head. This half circle should take 10 seconds.

Step 4

Exhale as you slowly lower your feet over the left shoulder, going to 4 inches above your left hand and continuing in a half circle to the left, taking 10 seconds.

Step 5

Heels extended, hold for five seconds once again in the cross position. The pelvis is tilted. Repeat in the opposite direction.

Helpful Hints

If your spine comes off the mat as you lower your legs in Steps 1 or 5, you may bend your knees slightly.

Keep your shoulders on your mat at *all* times during the five steps.

Keep your *heels extended* through this movement.

SPACE WALK

This is terrific for strengthening the lower back and abdomen.

It is not an exercise for a weak lower back. *Check with your doctor to see if there is any reason why you should not do this exercise.*

Lie on your back and place your hands palm down under your hips. Bend the knees, bringing

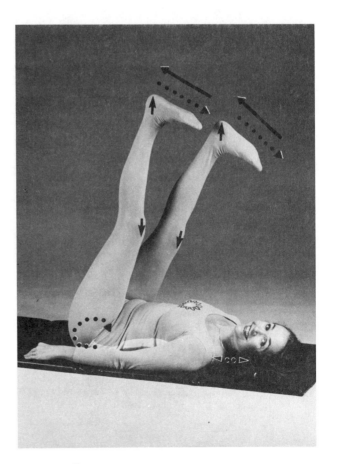

Space Walk

them to your chest; then straighten your legs. Your feet should be toward the ceiling.

Look up toward your feet; then *walk vigorously*, extending your heels and keeping the feet moving toward the wall behind you. Continue the movement, working up to 30 seconds. Your hips stay on the floor.

Lower your legs to the floor. Relax. Breathe normally throughout the exercise.

Remove your hands from beneath your hips and place them alongside your body. Repeat one more time.

Helpful Hints

If at first you are unable to straighten your legs, bend your knees slightly and keep working on Single Leg Raises with a belt or tie.

SIDE LEG LIFTS

These are two strong exercises for attacking the saddlebags of the outer thighs. The exercises are also good overall leg strengtheners. All leg raises improve the venous blood flow and help to avoid varicose veins.

Technique 1

As you lie on your left side, look down your body and see that the elbow, upper arm, chest, hip, and legs are in straight alignment.

Bend the left elbow and cup your head in your left hand. Again realign the elbow, rib cage, and hip. Place your right hand on the floor in front of you.

Tighten your seat and press your hips *forward*. Now flex your right foot and raise the right leg up approximately 8 to 10 inches. Look up to your right shoulder. Is your pelvis still pressed forward? Your foot should be kept flexed at all times.

Raise and lower your leg 20 times without pausing

Keep your shoulder perpendicular to the floor. Press your right hand to the floor for balance. Repeat on the opposite leg.

Technique 2

Line up your body as in Technique 1. Looking over your right shoulder for the alignment, inhale and raise the right leg in line with your shoulder and hips as you bend the right knee and draw it vigorously toward your right elbow and chest. Inhale and return your leg up toward the ceiling. Continue this powerful movement 10 to 20 times for each leg without pausing.

Helpful Hints

Because you are using weak thigh and hip muscles, the tendency will be to slouch backward. It's so much easier! So keep the pressure on yourself. *Tell yourself hips forward, legs in alignment with hips and shoulder.*

ALL SHOULDER WORK

The following all-shoulder-work exercises will increase your shoulder girdle mobility and strength. They will make an excellent foundation for flexibility and strength within postures. They firm the upper-back and chest muscles and aid in reducing round shoulders, dowager's hump, and arthritic and bursitis pain. Release of the stiffness in your shoulders will help your golf and tennis games.

Tense men and women reflect their tensions in muscles of this area, creating rigid and frozen chests

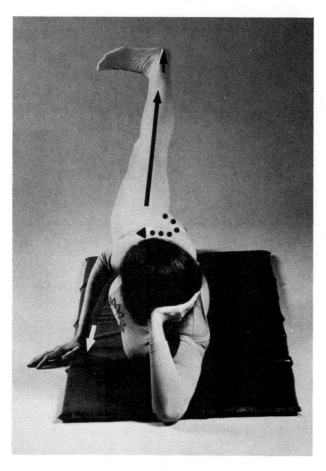

Side Leg Lifts

Lilias, Yoga, and Your Life

and shoulders. This rigidity affects the entire body alignment, which in turn affects your energy flow as well as your respiratory process.

ELBOW PULL

Stand with your feet 2 feet apart. Hands are on your hips, fingers pointing toward the navel.

Inhale, pulling your shoulders back as far as possible. The chest is now open. Lift the sternum.

Then exhale, pulling your elbows forward as far as possible and concaving your chest.

Slowly repeat this movement 8 times.

PUSH AWAY

Extend your arms evenly in front of you. Your arms are at shoulder height, your palms turned upward.

Inhale, then exhaling, extend your right arm and shoulder forward to its maximum. Pretend you are pushing against a wall with one arm and releasing the wall with the other. Keep the elbows straight.

Extend and release each arm 8 times.

HANDS UP

Stand with your feet 2 feet apart, arms at your sides, palms to the back wall.

Inhale and raise your elbows to shoulder level, fingertips pointing down to the floor.

Exhale and rotate your arms by using your shoulder girdle, lifting the forearms upward, fingertips toward the ceiling, upper arms still at shoulder level.

Inhale; then exhale. Return your hands to your sides. Make these three steps as one smooth motion. Repeat 10 times.

ROPE REACH

Stand or kneel, knees 2 feet apart. Extend your arms over your head as if holding a rope. Make two separate fists. Inhale and dynamically tense your right arm and reach upward as high as possible. Exhale, pulling down with your right arm with much resistance to the rope.

Repeat 10 to 15 times for each arm. Then relax your arms at your sides and shake out the tension.

CHICKEN WINGS

Start this position by standing with the feet two feet apart. Place your hands on your shoulders. Extend the elbows out from your hands on your shoulders. Extend the elbows out from your sides at shoulder level. Inhale.

Exhale slowly to 3 counts. Squeeze the shoulder blades together, back, and then down until your upper arms touch your side. Pause. Inhale.

Exhale. Continue the circle by drawing your elbows together toward the center until your elbows touch.

Inhaling, open the elbows up to your start position. Reverse the above process. Repeat 3 times in each direction.

TOWEL CLASP

Stand with your feet 2 feet apart. Clasp your towel, tie, or belt behind you. Your hands are 12 inches or hip-distance apart. Your fingernails are facing your buttocks muscles.

Inhale, lift the sternum, and shrug your shoulders back and down from your ears. Exhale and pull downward on your belt, rotating the eyes of your inner elbows toward your back until your arms are straight.

Relax your neck.

Inhale again; then exhale. Lift the arms up pulling down on your towel, thus pulling your shoulders down from your ears. Do not lean forward. Keep your pelvis tipped throughout the pose. Stand tall.

ANKLE CROSSOVER

Stand with your right foot crossed over your left. Lift the heel of your right foot and place your weight on your left foot. The ball of the right foot is for balance.

Clasp your hands behind you, fingers intertwined. Now straighten your elbows. Squeeze your shoulders together and down. Inhale.

Exhale and sway your arms to the right as your torso stretches to the left as far as possible. Your body weight is on the left foot. Hold for 3 seconds.

Inhale and then stretch your body in the other direction. Hold for 3 seconds and then exhale.

Change legs, cross left foot over the right. All the weight now is on the right foot. Repeat on opposite side.

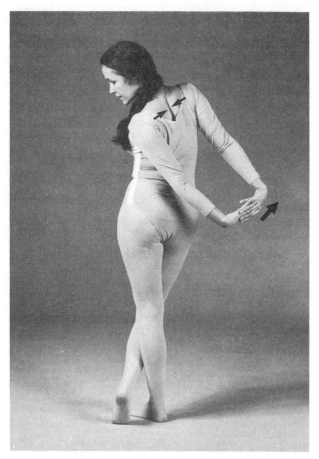

Ankle Crossover

two fists. Pull the shoulders down from your ears. This is your start position.

Inhale. Then, exhaling, simultaneously round your spine, bend the knees, and draw your fists together and drop the head between your upper arms.

Pause and inhale. Then, exhaling, continue emphasizing your cross-arm motion, bringing the right fist over the left elbow and left elbow over right fist. Hold.

Inhale, slowly returning to your start position. Knees straight, pelvis tucked.

Exhale, pressing your shoulders back. Squeeze the blades together. Think *tall* with the *top* of your head. Pause.

Repeat the complete series 4 to 8 times.

Be attentive to your breathing patterns.

TWO-ARMED LEMON SQUEEZE

With your arms out to the side in the T position pull your shoulders down from your ears.

Inhale and stretch your arms and hands out as far as possible. Feel them lengthen and the skin stretch. Hold to the count of 5.

Exhaling, bend your elbows and slowly draw both shoulder blades together as though you were squeezing a lemon between your shoulder blades. Hold for 5 seconds, then release. Repeat this squeeze-hold-release motion 3 to 5 times.

Helpful Hints

Do this movement with your arms, not by lifting your shoulders. Be sure to relax your neck.

HULK

Stand with feet 3 feet apart, toes straight ahead. Bend your elbows and extend them out to your sides. Elbows are at shoulder level and your hands make

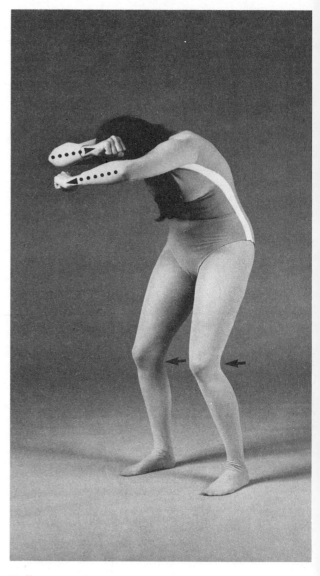

Hulk

Lilias, Yoga, and Your Life

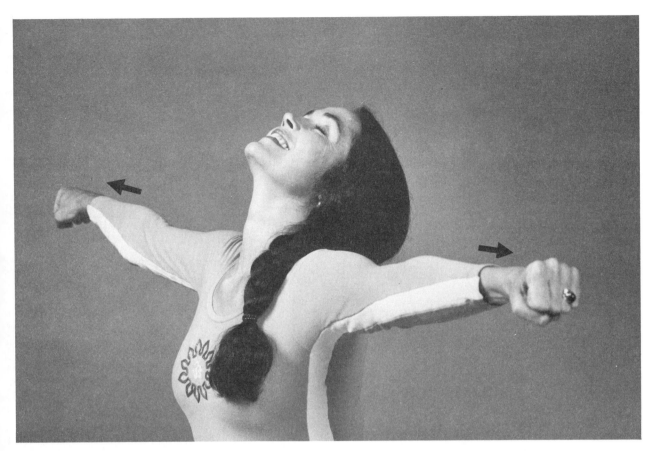

Arm Circles

ARM AND HEAD ROTATIONS

Here are two simple arm and head rotations easily done totally clothed and excellent for removing tension in the shoulders and neck area. They are also good for strengthening weak and flabby upper arms.

ARM CIRCLES

Place your arms in a T position, arms extended outward shoulder height. Make a fist with your hands. Tighten the elbows and muscles of your arms and make a tight, small, circular motion with your arms quite rigid. Do 15 circles in one direction, then 15 circles in the other.

Now make a large circle with your arms and repeat 15 in each direction. Allow your breathing to be natural and effortless.

HEAD ROLLS

Hold the arms quietly at shoulder height, and slowly drop your head back. Feel the back of your head squeeze against the raised muscles of your shoulders. Now smoothly and slowly make a circle with your head. Drop your chin to your throat, and, still inhaling, bring your right ear to your right shoulder. Then, exhaling, bring your left ear to your left shoulder and finally your head back. Repeat, going in the opposite direction. Make it a very smooth movement. Take care with breath sequence, and take your time!

Your arms should be out during the entire exercise. If your arms ache, that is good! (But *no* pain!) The ache simply tells you this is weak-muscle area and needs more work. Take at least two to three minutes to do this exercise.

Helpful Hints

Hold 2 cans of soup in each hand while doing this exercise if you wish to build a little more strength and endurance.

7

More Stepping Stones

Over the years I've watched my own classes grimace, clutch their backs, and groan as they plowed through the Sitback. I found that all this was eliminated once I took this exercise apart and understood its mechanics. It then became more effective, strengthening, challenging, and yet fun to do. It also seemed just as effective to do three Sitbacks, held for 15 to 30 seconds with arm movements, as the 20 succession situps of days gone by.

When the exercise is done in the following manner, you should feel no back pain or strain. The muscle tone will return quickly to the entire abdominal area, and you can count on a trim, tight stomach.

THE SITBACK

Sit with your knees bent, feet on the mat, and place your hands over the abdominal muscles. Now lean back to that point when you feel you are going to collapse. (This is called your balance point.)

In this balance point, feel beneath your hands what is happening as your abdominal muscle is working, holding the position for a half minute as you go through this checklist:

1. Does the muscle dome out, or does it stay flat?
2. Is the muscle quivering?
3. Can you feel it above or below your waist?
4. Do you feel back strain?
5. Do you feel other muscles working in your jaw, neck, shoulders, arms, and legs?
6. Is this position comfortable or uncomfortable to hold?

The purpose of this checklist is to increase your awareness. So be very accurate. Repeat the Sitback one more time.

More than likely you felt your abdomen dome outward. You also felt that it would not stay flat, that the muscle quivered, and that you felt it "catch" or tighten above your waist. Many students will feel lower-back strain.

The domed abdominal muscle means that it is unused and is depending too much on your lower back for support; therefore, you feel the back strain, or eventually back strain could be created. The quiver is firming tension and should be tolerated and held to become strong. After a few weeks, when your upper-abdominal muscles become stronger, you will feel this quivering strength travel to your lower abdomen. This is the firming tension that will flatten your stomach. Any pain in your lower back means you are doing the exercise incorrectly.

HOLLOW LAKE

Now let us combine the basic building block, Pelvic Tilt, and a new technique called Hollow Lake into your Sitback.

The Pelvic Tilt you are all familiar with from page 17. When Hollow Lake is done properly, the

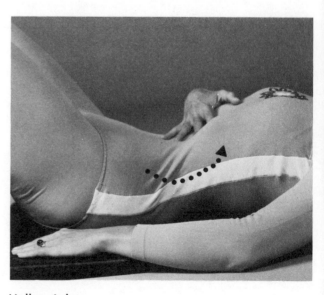

Hollow Lake

abdomen should feel hollow and smooth like a lake.

The Hollow Lake aids in elimination; it also strengthens the abdomen and lower back.

Lie on your mat. Bend your knees. Your knees are hip-distance apart.

Relax. Place your hands on your abdomen.

Inhale. Expand your chest, lift your breastbone.

Exhale; contract and tighten abdomen and pull shoulders down from your ears. Exhaling totally, tighten buttocks and sphincter muscle and simultaneously tilt your pelvis.

Do Not Inhale. Keep your mouth closed and do a mock inhalation. Refrain from breathing and smoothly draw in abdomen up toward your rib cage. When properly done, the abdominal muscles disappear to form a "hollow lake."

Hold this position as you let your breath flow deeply.

Repeat until the lake becomes one smooth procedure of action and breath.

Helpful Hints

There should be no gasping for breath. Practice will make this a smooth motion.

Relax your shoulders throughout.

At first use your hands to feel the lake.

Your pelvis stays tipped.

Your feet are not too close to your seat.

Try to clear as much air out of your lungs as possible, thus forming a vacuum that will enable you to draw your abdomen up.

At first it is natural to cough a little. Check the inclination to inhale.

Be sure you have learned to tighten your sphincter muscle from this lying-down position before continuing the exercise.

COMPLETE SITBACK

Now sit up, and we'll use the Pelvic Tilt and Hollow Lake within the Complete Sitback.

Sit on your mat with your knees bent, your heels about 2 feet from your buttocks. Your feet are flat on the floor, with your feet and knees 12 inches apart.

Place your hands on your knees; round your shoulders. Inhale, and then bring your chin toward your throat. Exhale as much as possible and do the Hollow Lake from a sitting position. Immediately contract the sphincter.

Then, once the abdomen goes hollow and you

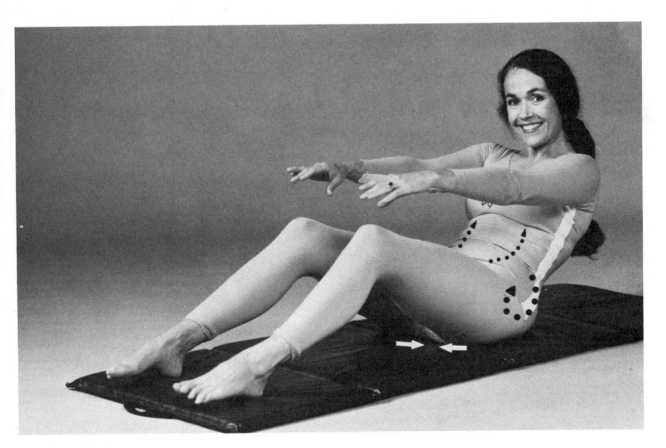

Complete Sitback, Step 3

More Stepping Stones

are breathing shallowly, release your hands and (breathing comfortably, abdomen pulled in) lean, with a rounded back, to your balance point.

At that moment of collapse, tilt the pelvis very, very firmly! Tighten the sphincter even more. The inner thighs are working; relax your shoulders and neck. Hold for 10 seconds, working up to 30 seconds. Smile!

Then come up to a sitting position.

Repeat 2 to 3 times. Then rest the abdomen completely. Lying down on your mat, take a few deep, Complete Breaths.

After a few weeks, you will become stronger. Therefore, start bringing your heels a little closer to your seat and repeat the entire exercise.

Advanced Arm Movements in Complete Sitback

When you feel comfortable and strong doing the preceding movements, proceed to add the arm movements.

Follow the directions for the Sitback, through the Hollow Lake and Complete Sitback. As you hold in your balance point, using the Pelvic Tilt, lift your arms directly out in front of you. Hold for 5 seconds.

Lift your arms up toward the ceiling. Hold for 5 seconds.

Cross your arms, elbows up toward ceiling. Hold for 5 seconds.

Raise your right arm; your left hand is to the floor. Hold for 5 seconds.

Extend both your arms out to the side in a V position; then cross them over your chest, apart. Cross over 3 times. Hold for 5 seconds. Lie down and relax.

Helpful Hints

Do all these arm motions smoothly without losing your hollow lake.

Keep the sphincter muscle locked throughout the exercise. This will add strength.

Remember to breath shallowly as you hold the lake.

Extend the arm movements from 5 to 10 seconds for more advanced work.

The rounded back will help activate your abdominal muscles.

Go over the checklist on page 32 again. With all the corrections you've learned, feel good about yourself and what your have accomplished.

ONE LEG FORWARD BEND

Sit. Place both hands around your right instep, with knee-cap pulled up. Heel extended. If you are working with a great deal of stiffness, place your hands around the calf.

Hold on to your instep (foot, ankle, calf) firmly. Inhaling, extend line of navel to sternum by pulling up from the waist; shoulders are pulled down from the ears.

Exhaling, rotate hips, and lead with the sternum as you stretch forward. Do the Shoulder Squeezes. (See pages 15–17.)

Bring your elbows down toward the floor; hands are on either side of the feet.

With each inhalation, *elongate the spine and rotate the hips*.

With each exhalation, advance toward your legs.

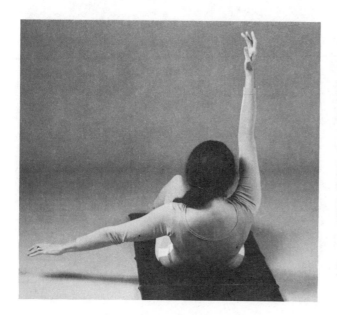

Advanced Arm Movements in Complete Sitback

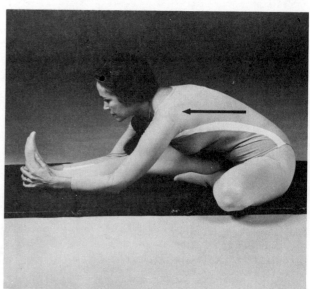

One Leg Forward Bend

Work very, very slowly toward your maximum edge. This entire procedure should take at least one minute, your breathing and body working together.

Come up slowly. Repeat with the opposite hip.

Helpful Hints

Keep your chin up and neck relaxed throughout all variations.

Remember to pull the thigh muscles out from under you *before* you start the posture. You will come down a half inch farther.

Remind yourself that what is important is not how far down you can get in the pose, but how well you apply the technique.

Do not hit your maximum edge of the forward bend within the first few seconds of the pose. Play your edge with your breathing and awareness.

Do not force yourself into the pose.

FORWARD LEG STRETCH

Before you start, correct the tendency for the bent left knee to drift out to the left as you are doing this stretch! For knee-cartilage safety, keep that bent knee in line with your left hip at all times.

Technique 1

Lie down on the mat. Bend both knees. Place the feet flat on the floor. Inhale. Exhaling, tilt the pelvis.

Inhale, extending the right heel toward the ceiling. Place both hands around your right calf. Exhale as you draw the right leg closer to your face by bend-

ing the elbows outward. Pull the shoulders down from your ears. The head stays on the mat.

Keep stretching the back of your leg by applying gentle leverage with both hands and working the stretch with three rhythmic breaths. Inhale as you extend the heel. Relieve the pressure slightly and exhale as you work the leg in closer. Keep the leg straight, kneecap pulled up. I'm not as interested in your coming close to your face with your leg as I am in your keeping your leg straight.

Return the left foot to the floor and repeat the entire procedure with your right leg.

Technique 2

Repeat Technique 1, but this time raise your face close to your kneecap. Play the edge of the stretch as you keep the heel extended. Inhale. Then, on your exhalation, work the knee closer to your face. Take three breaths; work your edge slowly.

ONE LEG FORWARD BEND WITH TWIST

Follow the directions for the One Leg Forward Bend (see page 34).

But this time, place the right elbow on the outside of your right knee. Clasp the right ankle with your right hand. The kneecap is pulled up; the foot is flat.

Place your left hand to the left big toe.

Inhale. Then, as you exhale, try to twist the upper torso through your arms. Continue working the twist more deeply by using your breathing. Inhale and hold at your edge. As you exhale, pull the

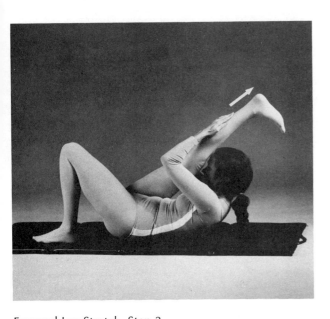

Forward Leg Stretch, Step 2

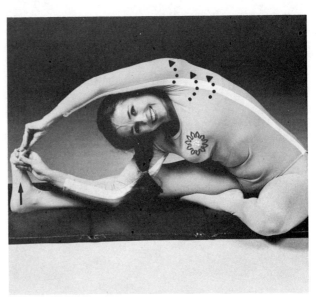

One Leg Forward Bend with Twist

More Stepping Stones

left shoulder back and turn the navel to the center.

Hold this pose for 10 to 30 seconds. Use your exhalation and leverage of the elbow and knee to aid this twist.

Release and repeat on opposite leg.

Helpful Hints

Keep looking under your arm as you hold the position.

Do not force your hand to the toe; just come as far as you can with no strain.

DANCER'S POSE

Notice that with a little practice, areas of the feet and ankles, which once felt separated and ungainly, will soon begin to move and act as one.

After you get the hang of it, try this movement a little faster. It should feel as if you're shooting energy out your feet and toes. Work up to 20 times with both legs.

Sitting on the floor, place your legs carefully into

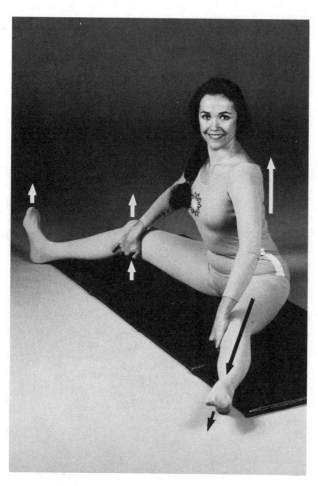

Dancer's Pose

a V position. Please do not strive to reach the maximum edge of the V at first. Feel the stretch but definitely *not* pain. Massage the inner thigh, knee, and calf if you are very tight.

Place your hands firmly on the inside of the knees, or place the fingertips on the floor close to the seat. Straighten your spine with the aid of the arms. Think *up* with the chest and chin and top of head.

Look down at your feet and heels and keep your heels glued to the floor. Bend both knees, flexing both feet, keeping spine straight. Hold for 5 seconds. Feel the bottom of your feet stretching.

Now straighten your knees; stretch the arches and feet. Reach with your toes (if you feel any foot or toe cramps, relax those muscles or give a quick massage) and contract the thigh muscles.

Repeat this bend-straighten movement 6 to 10 times. Make the movements smooth and hold each 3 to 5 seconds.

Repeat, but this time bend one leg as you straighten the other. Try this slowly at first and then speed the movement up, holding only 3 seconds.

Breathe comfortably throughout the exercise.

Helpful Hints

Stretch the legs out in a V against the wall before doing this exercise.

Take special care when *placing* the legs in a V. It is extremely easy to overstretch the ligaments of the inner thigh. Once overstretched, they can take many months to heal.

As you speed up the movement, remember to keep your heels glued to the mat.

Do not let your legs roll inward during the exercise.

KNEES SIDE TO SIDE

A simple but effective warmup for your spine.

Step 1

Lie on your mat. Bend both knees to your chest. Arms are in a T position. Pull your shoulders down from the ears. Roll side to side with your knees 3 to 6 times in a smooth movement.

Step 2

Inhale. Then as you exhale, bring both knees together underneath your right arm down on the mat. You will now hold this pose for 30 seconds.

Inhale and reach with the fingertips and stretch the muscles across your chest. As you relax, press your left shoulder to the mat gently.

As you hold the knees to the right, breathe rhythmically 3 to 6 times. Inhale. Then stretch and lengthen. Then exhale and press the shoulders to the mat.

Release, bringing both knees to the chest and repeating to the left, holding for 30 seconds, working with the breath.

Helpful Hints

Do not force your shoulder to the mat; let your breath take it down.

SIDE ROCK AND ROLL

This movement warms up and stretches the muscles on either side of the spinal column. It's fun. It tests your coordination.

Technique 1

Sit on your mat, hands holding on to crossed insteps.

Round the spine. Inhale; then exhale. Roll backward from your right hip back to your right shoulder. Then roll up to a sitting position 3 times to the right.

Now roll down and back up 3 times on the left.

Technique 2

Follow the above directions, but this time roll from right hip to left shoulder and then go from left hip to right shoulder. Repeat 3 times.

INTERMEDIATE CROSSED ANKLE ROCK AND ROLL

Step 1

Sit with ankles crossed, holding on to your instep. Hold onto insteps throughout pose.

Inhale. Then as you exhale, pull the stomach to inhale and lift the sternum; sit tall. As you exhale, round the spine and bring the forehead to the floor in front of you. Your buttocks stay on the floor. Hold this position, applying gentle pressure with your hands downward to the instep. Now bring the right shoulder up to your right ear, release, and repeat 3 times for each shoulder. Then, inhale and raise both shoulders; exhale and pull them down from ears.

Step 2

Inhale and sit up, then roll back on your mat, holding on to the instep. Exhale as you bring the toes behind your head.

Hold the toes to the floor firmly, bending both knees and letting your lower back relax. Push your

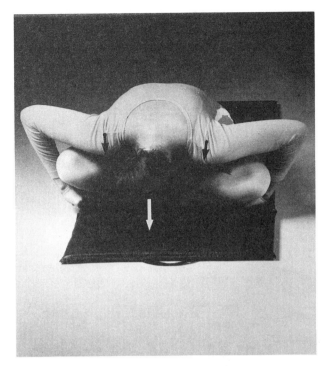

Intermediate Crossed Ankle Rock and Roll (Step 1)

shoulders into the mat as you hold, relaxing for 15 seconds. Then start to extend the heels, lifting the perineum (crotch) toward the ceiling. Concentrate on breathing slowly as your work your legs straight, extending both heels and raising kneecaps.

Step 3

To lower your body, bend both knees to the chest. Inhale and round the spine as you let your but-

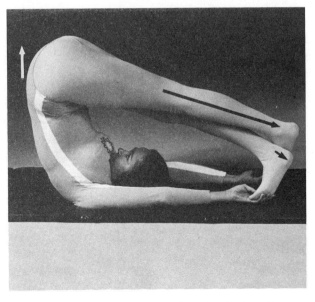

Intermediate Crossed Ankle Rock and Roll (Step 2)

More Stepping Stones

tocks roll to the mat. Still holding on to the toes, pull your heels against the back of the thighs; use this leverage to swing the knees forward and then down to your mat. This motion will bring you up to your sitting pose.

Exhale, again bringing your forehead to the mat. Repeat this warmup 3 times. Then reverse ankles and repeat.

Helpful Hints

Remember, to get more stretch, inhale as you elongate the back and raise the hips. Exhale and extend the heels, pulling your toes in toward your head.

Make this a coordinated rhythmic motion as you rock.

Do not cross arms.

LUNGE WARMUP

A dynamic thigh strengthener, the Lunge Warmup tones and firms the buttocks and removes unwanted fat from the thighs. Excellent exercise to prepare the thighs, hips, and ankles for the rigors of skiing. This is difficult for beginners, so I have broken this Lunge Warmup into 3 steps.

The Dancer's Pose is suggested as a preliminary exercise.

Step 1

Stand with your feet 4 feet apart. Pivot on the heel of your right foot, turning it outward and left foot in.

Inhale, bending the right knee directly over the right foot. As you exhale, lean forward and place your hands on the mat in front of you.

Hold this position for 5 to 10 seconds. Breathe shallowly, letting the muscles of the left leg stretch out. Bring the outer rim of your left foot to mat. The knee should be straight.

Now inhale deeply. Then exhale as you push down on your hands and spring up into a standing position. Repeat once again on the right leg. Then twice on the left leg.

Step 2

Do as above, but this time use the hands less and the thighs more. And instead of holding, pause briefly; then come up so you are now starting a rhythm.

Step 3

Now go through Step 2 without using hands. The rhythm is important and makes it easier. Keep your heels flat on the floor and hold your torso as erect as possible. Work up to 5 to 10 repetitions without stopping. Rest. Then repeat 5 to 10 more times.

Helpful Hints

Look down and recheck to see that your bent knee is in alignment with your foot. Allowing the knee to drift to either side puts undue strain on knee cartilage.

INCLINED PLANE

This posture firms and develops the pectoral muscles, tightens and firms the seat, and expands the chest for easier breathing. It strengthens the wrists and the lower arms and "oils" the shoulders. It is an excellent warmup for tennis or golf.

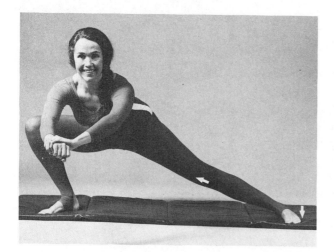

Lunge Warmup

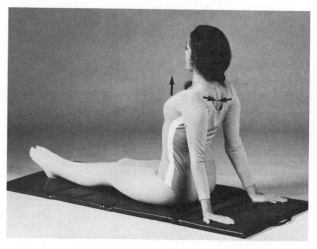

Inclined Plane (hands behind you)

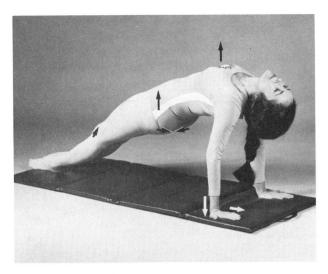

Inclined Plane (hips higher)

Sit with your legs outstretched.

Place your hands behind you on the mat with fingers facing the wall to your back. Squeeze shoulder blades together.

Swallow. Drop your head back.

Inhale; then as you exhale, lift the hips off the floor. Come to the highest point, or "top," of the pose.

Then pull the kneecaps up. Tighten the buttocks; squeeze the shoulders together; extend the chest. Lift the breastbone. Make your body as straight as possible, pushing the heels into the floor.

Hold. Then think about lifting your hips a half inch higher!

Continue breathing and hold for 10 to 20 seconds.

Exhale. Lower your bottom to the floor.

Helpful Hints

Remember the building block of squeezing the shoulder blades.

Relax the feet if your toes cramp together at the top of the pose.

Rotate on your heels placing the feet in a straight line when it comes time for the side variations.

Swallow before you drop your head back, *not* during this motion.

Variation 1

Repeat the above procedure. Come to the top of the pose.

Slowly raise the right leg; the foot can be flexed or pointed.

Hold for 5 seconds; keep breathing; don't let your body collapse! Release.

Lower your leg and repeat on the opposite side.

Variation 2

Come into the top of the pose. Then turn onto right hand and lift your left shoulder up toward the ceiling. Place the left hand on the left thigh. Keep your head in alignment with your spine. Turn the feet to the left to form a straight line.

Then, exhaling, drop your right hip to a few inches from the ground.

Sink deeply into the right shoulder. There is a "hanging" feeling within the shoulder.

As you inhale, come up to the side inclined-plane position.

Turn and repeat on the opposite side.

Variation 3

Go into the top of the pose; turn to the right; lift the left shoulder up to the ceiling; tighten the buttocks; pull the kneecaps up. Turn your feet to the right to form a straight line.

Inhaling, raise your left arm up close to the left ear. Keep the left arm very straight.

Feel the stretch down the side of the ribs and the hip.

Inhale and lift the left ribs and hip a little higher to the ceiling.

Hold for 5 seconds. Taking a deep breath, turn and repeat on the opposite hand.

Helpful Hints

Exercise on a non-skid surface.

Pay attention to the side-pivotal movement of the feet.

Line up the feet in one straight line, or heel to toe, as you go from side to side.

PUSHUP 1

This exercise and the two following are for those with weak upper-arm and chest muscles.

Place the hands and knees on the mat. The palms of the hands are on the floor directly beneath the shoulders. The knees are directly beneath the hips. Turn your toes under.

Inhale; then exhaling, lower the chest and chin to the floor. The collarbone is in line with the thumbs. The chest is pressed to the floor. Hold for 5 seconds, breathing shallowly. The elbows are close to the body.

Inhale; then exhaling, raise the chest off the floor. Back to the mat pose. In a few weeks you will be able to lift your chest with a degree of strength. Then add the leg action.

PUSHUP 2

In the mat pose, lift the right leg up. Inhale; then, exhaling, lower the chin and chest to the floor, and gently press the chest into floor. Elbows should be close to the body. Hold for 5 seconds, breathing shallowly. On the exhalation, straighten your elbows, spine arched, heels extended toward ceiling.

With leg extended repeat 3 times.

Repeat, using the opposite leg.

PUSHUP 3

Lie on your abdomen. Bend the knees and bring your feet up toward the ceiling. Place the hands parallel to the breastbone, elbows close to body.

Your face is toward the mat. As you tighten the buttocks muscles and tilt the pelvis, press your palms into the mat. Exhaling, raise yourself up to an absolutely straight line. The knees stay on the mat.

Inhale and lower yourself, parallel to the floor. Keep the shoulders squeezed, trying not to hunch over.

Exhaling, push down on heels of hands, and lift back up to a straight line.

Repeat 3 to 6 times.

Helpful Hints

Keep your pelvis slightly tipped to keep your stomach pulled up.

Relax your neck and chin area.

Place toes on floor if bringing your feet up toward the ceiling is at first too difficult.

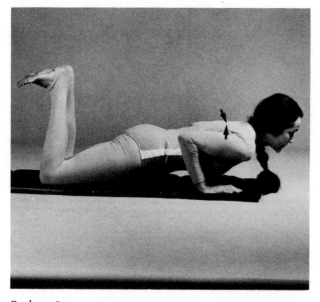

Pushup 3

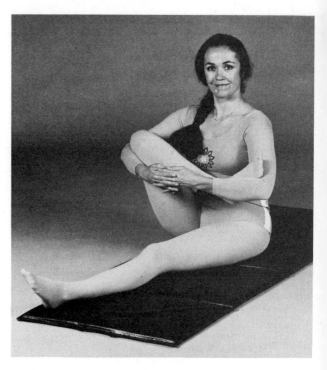

Rock-a-Baby, or Hip Rock

ROCK-A-BABY, OR HIP ROCK

This exercise brings increased circulation to the hip and leg area. A good warmup for all athletes.

Sore and stiff joints develop for many different reasons. (Read chapter 13, "Back Talk.") Rock-a-Baby brings a little "oil" to the muscles, ligaments, and cartilage of the universal joint of the hip. Also, the entire foot and ankle (usually encased in a shoe) receive special attention with a gentle, oblique stretch. The spine and lower-back muscles lengthen and warm up gradually. This is an exercise that feels really good.

Sit on the floor, legs straight out in front of you. Reach down and bring your right foot into the crook of your bent left elbow. (Look down and check to see that the position of your foot is correct, as in the photo.)

Then reach around your right knee with the right arm and firmly clasp the hands together. Then as you exhale, gently pull the leg toward the chest. Repeat 3 times.

After you have warmed up the hip socket with this press-release motion, slowly rock your leg in a side-to-side motion for 30 seconds.

When the muscles feel warmer and looser, increase the stretch of the back by sitting up straighter. Continue rocking your leg from side to side; breathing is shallow and comfortable.

Repeat the exercise on the opposite leg.

Lilias, Yoga, and Your Life

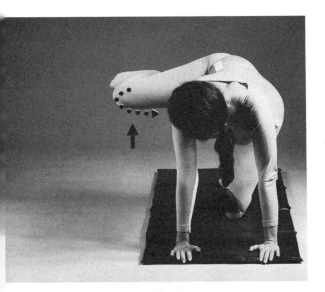

Hydrant

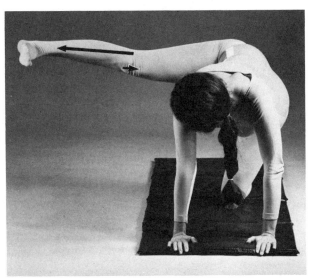

Hydrant (leg parallel to floor)

HYDRANT

The Hydrant is absolutely perfect for those who would like to reach and firm those stubborn fatty areas of the outer and inner thighs. It is an excellent hip warmup for the runner.

Start by working on completing this exercise once with each leg. (It should take at least 30 seconds to do each side.) Then, in a few weeks' time, work up to completing the exercise 3 times each leg, taking 1 minute for each side.

Kneel on the mat, placing your hands directly beneath the shoulders. Knees are together, parallel with your hips. Inhale, then as you exhale, bend the right knee; drop the spine, and draw your knee to your nose. Inhale, raise the chin, arch your spine and raise the right heel behind you up toward the ceiling. Pause; then bend the right knee and look over your right shoulder to the right thigh. (Note photo.) Adjust the right bent leg so that the upper thigh is parallel to the floor so that you cannot see your right foot.

Hold this position breathing shallowly. (If you are having trouble holding your leg up, it is best not to persist. In a few more weeks, when your body is more flexible and strong, you can continue.)

Take a few more deep breaths as you move and attain the correct position.

Now slowly draw the right knee in toward your right shoulder. Do not drop the right hip. Try and lift it higher.

Take more breaths while holding. Flex the right foot.

From this position, straighten out the right leg; extend your heel. The foot is flat. Keep looking at the leg, making sure it stays parallel with the floor. Hold for two more breaths.

Then lift your chin up, arch the spine. Right heel up toward the ceiling.

Now, repeat the same procedure on the left leg. When finished, rest, sitting on your heels, with arms alongside legs, forehead to the floor. Relax.

Helpful Hints

Do *not* bend your arm or lean sideways to get the leg up.

Do the variations once you are familiar with the pose. When the leg is out to the side and parallel to the floor, bring the toe down to the floor; then bring it back to the side parallel position.

SKY DIVER

This strengthens and tones the seat; it also helps remove any fat from back of thighs and seat.

Lie on the mat on your stomach, arms directly out in front of you, shoulders-width apart.

Inhale deeply; then exhale, tip the pelvis, and then firmly lift both legs off the floor. Keep the seat tight.

Inhale and lift the arms and chest and ribs, and raise the chin so your head is between the upper arms. Breathe shallowly.

Now raise the head even higher and spread your feet away apart and lift and spread arms out in a T position. Push the heels of your hands into the floor on either side of you. Keep the pelvis tilted as you lift your legs and upper chest and head. Ask yourself, "What am I doing?" Flying through the air, of

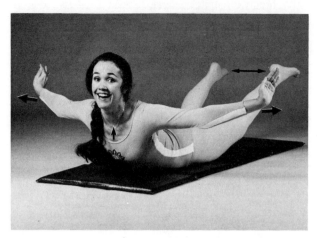

Sky Diver

course! Fly for 15 seconds. Feel the weightlessness of your body; then relax. Turn and rest your cheek on the mat and take one Complete Breath.

Repeat once more.

SPINAL WARMUP 1

This and the two following warmups condition the upper back and abdomen. They also stimulate your nervous system.

Lie face down on the mat with your feet together. Place your forehead on the mat and look down the front of your body. Your feet should be together. Arms are alongside your body, palms turned up. Raise your forehead, nose, and chin off the mat. You should feel a gentle pressure where your neck and the back of your head meet.

Inhale; contract buttocks muscles; lift chest off the mat, using your abdominal muscles (no arms or hands); pull the shoulders down and squeeze your shoulder blades together.

Hold your breath as long as you comfortably can.

Exhale, slowly releasing the lower chest and shoulders; tuck in your chin, nose and forehead to the mat. Relax. Repeat 3 times.

SPINAL WARMUP 2

This conditions the upper back as well as the cervical and dorsal curves. It also relieves tension in the shoulders and holds the vertebrae in alignment.

As you place the forehead on the mat, the arms are alongside the body, feet together. Bring the arms behind your back; clasp the hands together, interlocking your fingers; straighten the elbows.

Look down the front of your body. Then raise your forehead, nose and chin. Inhale. Raise the shoulders and chest; contract your buttocks muscles. Raise your arms up and back. Keep your elbows straight; squeeze the shoulder blades together. Hold for 3 seconds.

Exhaling, lower your chest, shoulders and arms, and tuck in chin; lower your chin, nose, and forehead to the mat. Relax and repeat.

SPINAL WARMUP 3

Lie on your stomach. Extend your arms over the head; palms of your hands on the floor 6 inches apart, arms straight. Contract your seat muscles. Tilt the pelvis. Inhale, raise your head, and walk the hands in 2 inches toward the body. Hold this position. Then walk the hands in a few more inches. Hold. Breathe comfortably. Then walk them in enough to just barely raise the navel off the floor, but *no* higher. Hold pose. Raise your right arm up, relaxing shoulders and keeping your neck free from tension. Breathing comfortably, hold 5 seconds. Then lower your arm and walk down slowly as you come up. The entire movement should take 30 seconds.

Helpful Hints

Look down the front of your body to get the feeling of a free, elongated neck.

Feel your legs extending back.

Use your breathing to aid in strengthening your control with the up-and-down motion.

Place a rolled towel or small pillow beneath your hips and pubic bone if needed for added comfort.

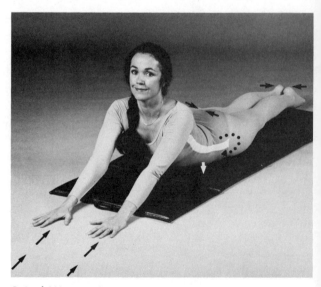

Spinal Warmup 3

Lilias, Yoga, and Your Life

LOCUST WARMUP

I realize that "sagging bottom" is frustrating but it is absolutely curable! People who sit all day should pay special attention to these exercises.

The largest part of your bottom is just one muscle, the gluteus maximus. As this muscle becomes weak through inactivity, it drops and makes a bulge on the upper thigh. With these Locust warmups, you will focus particularly on this muscle and get it working.

If at first the buttocks (not lower back) become a little sore, it is a good sign. It means you are getting into an area within your body that needs some work. Stay with it. In a few weeks' time this discomfort will be gone.

If these exercises are performed faithfully, the seat muscle and hamstrings will become higher, firmer, and stronger. A hamstring is any of the tendons that form the boundaries of the ham, or hollow of the knee.

Technique 1

Lie on your abdomen; place the hands alongside the body, palms down. The chin should be on the floor, feet together. (This is the basic start position of the Locust.)

Inhale through the nose; then exhaling, lift the right leg up toward the ceiling; hold your breath and position for 3 seconds. Keep both hips firmly on the mat. Repeat 3 times for each leg. Rest; then repeat 3 more times. (If the positioning of the chin to the floor makes your upper neck uncomfortable, turn your cheek to the side.)

Technique 2

Lie on your abdomen; make two fists with your hands. Place arms alongside body. It is very important that you keep the inner part of the arms and elbows on the floor. Have your hands make two fists, thumbs to mat. If this maneuver feels painful, stop and place the palms flat alongside your body. You can add the arm position later as you become more flexible.

Inhale. Exhale and come onto knees bringing your knees to your fists. Smoothly raise the right leg. (Note photo.) Breathe shallowly as you hold this position 3 to 5 seconds. Here hips *do* come off the mat. Don't let the leg sway to the left. Keep the hips parallel. Slowly, lower the leg to the floor, returning to the knees. Repeat the entire exercise with the opposite leg.

Then lie flat, bringing your arms out from under your torso.

Make a pillow of your hands. Relax the entire body, feet well apart. Take 3 deep breaths. When you become familiar with the movements, do 3 leg lifts each side.

Helpful Hints

Perform the movements smoothly.

Use the buttocks muscles and entire arm for lift.

Do not do this movement in a quick or jerky manner.

Do not get discouraged if at first your leg feels like 10 tons.

STAR

The Star releases tension and soothes the lower back.

Sit on the mat. Bend your knees and place the soles of your feet together. Bring the feet out about 16 to 24 inches *away* from the groin.

Round your back, lean forward, and slip the hands on top of each instep, elbows on the floor. Then place the hands on the tips of your feet, touching the toenails.

Inhale; then exhaling, relax your shoulders and buttocks muscles. Inhale and exhale again, gently pulling the head toward your feet. Hold for 15 to 30 seconds. Suggest to your body that it relax during the exercise.

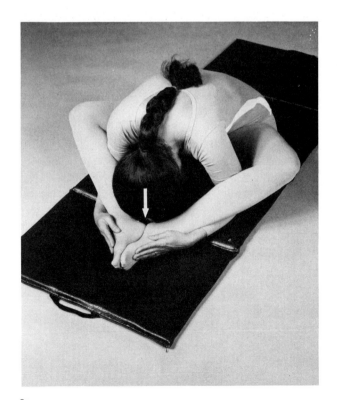

Star

HALF-MOON STANDING POSE

Here is a stretch directed to the midsection, for the waist and hips and upper arm.

Stand with feet 3 feet apart. Toes are forward. Bring your left arm around and rest it in the curve of your lower back. Fingers will protrude a few inches.

Place the right hand on top of your head. Then, lift your hand 6 inches.

Look to the inside of the right elbow. Be sure to point the elbow toward the ceiling.

Inhale and lift up; then exhaling, stretch to the left.

Keep looking at the inside of the right arm. Your elbow is up toward the ceiling. Do *not* lean forward. Hold for 5 seconds, breathing shallowly.

Inhale and slowly stand. Repeat on the opposite side.

Helpful Hints

Go slowly. Do one stretch on each side. Then after a few days work up to 3 each side. This is a stronger exercise than you think.

Pretend you are doing the Half-Moon against the wall.

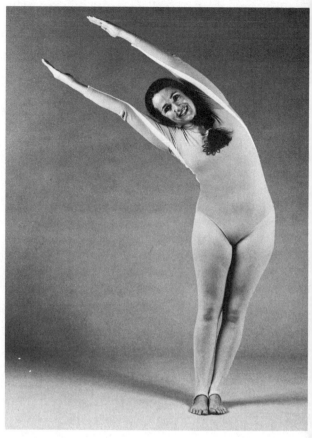

Standing Side to Side Pose

STANDING SIDE-TO-SIDE POSE (NITAMBASANA)

This is an especially good stretch for the sides of your body; and it's a terrific warmup.

Stand with the feet 12 inches apart.

Raise your arms up over your head lifting up out of your rib cage; elbows straight, pulling the arms back behind your ears. The palms of the hands face each other, wrists straight.

Inhale; then exhaling, stretch slowly to the right. Continue until you start to lean forward. Go no farther. Hold just *behind* your maximum edge of stretch, breathing shallowly. Pull the stomach in! Pull the shoulders back. Hold for 5 seconds.

Inhale and slowly return to the center.

Repeat on the opposite side.

In a few weeks, work up to 3 each side.

RAG DOLL

Here's a nice warmup to relax the body.

Stand with the feet together, drop your chin forward and relax your arms, and round your back. Slowly to the count of 10 seconds, lean forward in a very relaxed manner. Your face is relaxed, arms hang limply, neck is totally relaxed, not helping to hold up the head. By the last count of 10, you should be totally in your Standing Forward Bend. Hold for 5 seconds, breathing comfortably. Let your cheeks flow over your eyes.

Then to the count of 10, come up slowly from your Rag Doll by reversing the above process. The spine is rounded. Let your head be the very last to lift as you reach the count of 10. Repeat 3 times.

In all the standing poses, I suggest that your feet be bare and that you use a line on your floor. I have taped some black tape 3 inches from the wall and a 4½-foot line in the center of my room. This line helps me to become aware of my own foot and body alignment. Many of the following standing poses ask you to begin by placing your right foot at a right angle and to turn your left foot inward. (Note photo.) The ability to do this does not begin with the feet, but originates in the hip joint and the ligaments and tendons surrounding it. The degree of outward turn depends on the condition of the muscles involved in the outward leg rotation and the individual student's pelvic construction. The turning starts at the hip joint, then goes down through the bones and muscles of your thighs to your knees and then to your feet.

Many of the following poses ask you to have your feet 3 to 4 feet apart. This distance will vary (1) with the posture and (2) according to your height. If I say your feet should be 3 feet apart, but you are 5'9" and 3½ feet brings more balance to your pose, then, yes, adjust your feet. To keep your balance as you adjust your feet, slide the front leg forward while keeping your weight steady on your back, or anchor, leg.

When you raise your arms up into the T position, really *stretch* your arms right out to your fingertips. Keep your wrists straight and look down your arms. See if they are in line with your shoulders and if your shoulders are *pulled* down from your ears.

If you feel tension in the lower back during or after the pose, increase the pressure on your back (downward) leg or see if you have slouched forward.

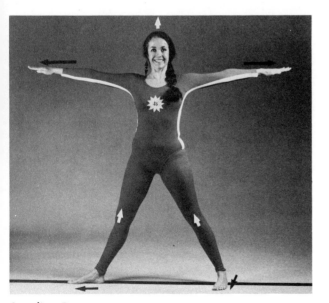

Standing Pose

8
Standing Poses

Remind yourself to think *upward* within the hips, spine, and then the tip of your head. Rest in between your standing poses.

The standing poses develop endurance, stamina, coordination, strength, and discipline. You cannot think of business matters or the laundry list if you are paying close attention to these *dynamic* poses. As never before, you should experience an inner awareness and body control.

I used to tease my TV classes by telling them that this type of toe-foot coordination is a great sign of intelligence!

The exercise will not lead to enlightenment, but it is amusing to try, and it *will* keep you in touch with your feet. It also reminds us that all standing poses need to be built on a firm platform of the feet.

Here is the technique.

Stand directly on the floor.

Look down at your feet and line up feet with the line on the floor. Toes 3 inches apart, heels 3 inches apart. Place your weight on the right side of your feet; then roll the weight toward both heels and the balls of the feet.

Now roll a slow circle to the right 3 times, then 3 times to the left. When you are done, feel if the weight is evenly distributed over the soles of the feet. Lift up all toes and lace them lightly on the floor like feathers.

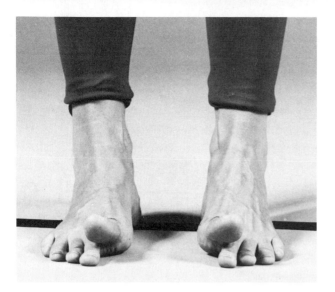

Standing Pose (big toe up)

Now raise up just the big toe, pressing the other four toes into the floor. Hold for 5 seconds. Relax.

Then press the big toe to the floor; lift up the other 4 toes. Hold for 5 seconds; relax.

Rest all the toes on the floor *lightly*. Feel new awareness between the heels and the balls of the feet.

To strengthen arches, walk around barefoot on the balls of your feet when possible.

STANDING POSE (TADASANA)

Stand with the feet 3 inches apart. Look down and *check* the feet. Are the toes 3 inches apart? Are the heels 3 inches apart, and in a straight line? Place your weight on the outer rim of both feet; then roll the weight lightly inward to evenly distribute the weight over the sole of the foot.

Now pull the kneecaps up and observe what has happened. You have "energized" your thighs and hip area. This little movement has caused the thighs to contract and the pelvis to tilt. Now tilt the pelvis consciously and lift the sternum.

Think *tall*, as if you have a small braid on the top of your head and it's being pulled upward. The neck is relaxed and free, the shoulders are down and gently back, and the arms hang in a relaxed manner.

TRIANGLE POSE (TRIKONASANA)

This posture means intense, extended triangular stretch to the sides, and that's *just* what happens! This tones the muscles of the legs and hips, stretches

and develops the intercostal muscles of the rib cage, relieves backache, and strengthens your neck. It also relieves menstrual cramps.

If you breeze through Triangle Pose, you can be sure you are not doing it correctly!

Step 1

Stand with the legs 3 feet apart, heels on the line. As you pivot on right heel lift the toes up on the right foot, rotating your right leg and placing the foot on the line. (The line splits the foot down the center.) Lift the toes of the left foot, rotating and pivoting your left foot inward 3 inches. Now rotate your inner thighs outward to keep the hips straight ahead. Raise both arms into your T position. Pull the shoulders down from the ears. Raise the kneecaps.

Step 2

Inhale and lift up the rib cage. Leading with the right arm, slide sideways to your right as you keep the arms parallel to the standing line.

Step 3

Then when you can go no farther place the right hand where it meets the right leg. Pull the kneecaps up; tighten the buttocks. Now look up to the thumb of the left hand and *think upward*. Inhale and extend your left hand higher from within the shoulder socket. Exhaling, rotate the navel and sternum toward the center of the room.

In Step 3 the feeling would be one of "upness" and correct body alignment, as if you're doing the posture against the wall. In fact, to aid yourself in correcting your body balance, place yourself against a wall and go through Steps 1–3.

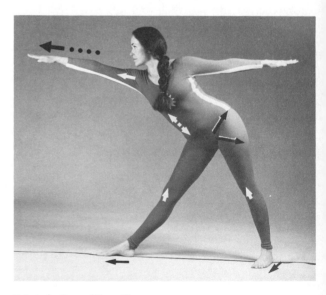

Triangle Pose (Step 2)

Lilias, Yoga, and Your Life

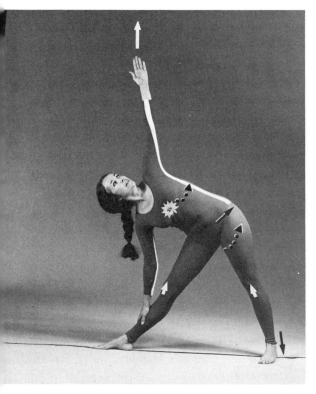

Triangle Pose (Step 3)

Helpful Hints

If you feel too much strain or stress in your back leg (anchor), do this pose briefly. Rotate the left hip forward just ½ inch to release this discomfort. Hold, relax, take a deep breath, and then slowly return the hip back to that point that is *behind* that feeling of too much strain or stress. This would be called playing the edge of your stretch.

As I learned this pose, I found it helpful to place a box or a large book alongside my right foot and then once again go to Step 3.

Place your hand on the book and concentrate on elongating (flattening) the side of the rib cage. Inhale and elongate; exhaling, continue the stretch.

Step 4

As you continue working with the pose, slowly work the hand down toward the right ankle. Turn from your ear to bring your chin in line with the shoulders as you look up to the thumb of your right hand. Repeat on left side.

Helpful Hints

Place the heels 3 inches out from the wall when you use the wall for practice. Remember the back leg is the anchor of all standing poses. See that the outer rim of the anchor foot is flat to the floor and kneecaps pulled up.

I suggest you can occasionally release the right hand that was on the lower leg, bend the right elbow and place the arm up on your lower back. This gesture keeps you honest. You want very little weight on that right hand because you want the upper body to do the work!

LATERAL ANGLE POSE

All standing poses are terrific for helping to make a shapely leg. They will help to fill in skinny thighs and to reduce fat on the hips.

Step 1

Stand with feet 4 feet apart, heels on the line, arms in the T position in line with your shoulders. Pivot on the right heel, placing the right foot on the line; then rotate and pivot on the left heel, turning your left foot in slightly. Now bend the right knee until the thigh and calf form a right angle. Your right thigh is parallel to the line.

Step 2

Inhale deeply; then exhale as you glide to the right, extending the right arm and rib cage. You are still over the line. Inhale and elongate the trunk diagonally. Exhaling, place the pads of the fingertips of your right hand on the outside by the side of the right foot. The right armpit is touching the outer side of your right knee. Look down and check to see that the right bent knee is directly in line with your foot.

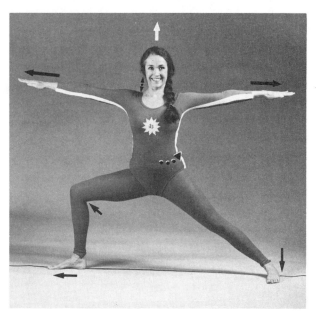

Lateral Angle Pose (Step 1)

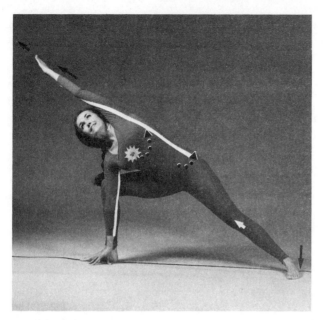

Lateral Angle Pose (Step 4)

Step 3

Now place your left hand around the outside of the left rib cage, thumb facing forward. Inhale. As you exhale, let the left hand pull the rib cage and left shoulder back. Navel and trunk are rotating forward toward the center of your room. Keep this rhythmical breathing going for 3 breaths, working your shoulder gently back and trunk turning.

Step 4

Touch the left hand to your left ear; then continue straightening the left arm. The left upper arm will now be close to your left ear. The head is in a straight line with the spine.

As you hold, with arms over the head for 3 more breaths, feel your skin, ribs, and spine being stretched. Pull your abdomen in and keep reaching, lifting, and lengthening as you hold. Exhale as you then straighten your right leg. Return to basic standing pose.

Repeat entire procedure to the left.

Helpful Hints

Throughout this movement take special care to be sure your bent knee is directly in line with your foot. If not, you are risking straining the cartilage of your knees.

As you become more confident in this pose, place the entire palm of your hand to the floor.

The power of this pose starts from the rim of your anchor (back) leg.

SHIELD

The Shield works the upper-thigh muscles and seat.

Work your way through Steps 1 and 2 in your Lateral Angle Pose, but instead of keeping the knee at a right angle, bend the knee farther forward so the right knee is now over your toes. The right heel stays glued to the floor.

Inhale as you extend the right arm, keeping it parallel to the floor line. Exhaling, place the tip of your middle right-hand finger in front of the instep of your right foot. The palm is flat and facing forward. No weight is to be placed on this middle finger. The hand is just decoration. Let the muscles of your upper thigh do all the work. Your body forms a strong shield.

Then lift the left arm directly up toward the ceiling. The palm is turned toward the center and is absolutely flat. Fingers together. Hold for 10–15 seconds, breathing comfortably. Inhale; then exhale.

Straighten the right knee and come up to your standing pose.

Repeat the pose on your left side.

Helpful Hints

The finger that touches the floor is not to support any sort of weight—no white fingertips!

Try this pose with heels 3 inches away from the wall. Let your body just graze the wall. This is just to give you a feeling of straightness.

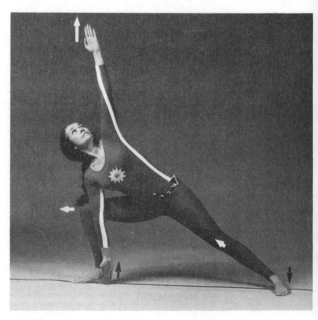

Shield

Lilias, Yoga, and Your Life

COBRA (BHUJANGASANA)

The Cobra pose is an extremely healthful spinal posture. In the full posture, the body resembles this hooded snake, its head back, ready to strike.

It is both maintenance and tonic for the entire nervous system, with deep muscles of the back alternately contracted and relaxed, thus helping to prevent backache.

The Cobra brings increased blood circulation into both the front and back areas of the spine, which ordinarily are difficult to reach. It gives back to the spine the elasticity so often lost with age and tension.

Abdominal muscles are tightened and organs of elimination are toned, due to pressure in the pelvic area.

The muscles, vertebrae, and ligaments of the spinal system have a balanced relationship, where each should carry its designated share of the work. When this delicate system becomes unbalanced, the other parts of it pick up an unnatural share of the workload. This exercise can help restore the natural balance.

The Cobra also firms the bust, neck, and chin, and is said to increase circulation to the prostate, ovaries, uterus, and gonads.

In the older books on Hatha Yoga, there is much attention given to arching your *entire* spine in Cobra. However, over the years, we've all seen too much lower-back discomfort and compression start due to doing the Cobra in this manner. My personal rule of thumb is *no pain, no discomfort, no vertebrae compression* to the lower back while in any pose. Keeping the navel just lightly to the floor will safeguard your lower back. Also tipping your pelvis will keep the lower back from overdoing this arch.

The Cobra is definitely possible for the beginning student, but it is also extremely difficult to do well, and therefore challenges the expertise of the intermediate student.

9

Other Postures and Poses

Lie on your abdomen on the mat, feet together. Place the heels of your hands on the mat approximately 2 inches above the collarbone; elbows are bent and close to the body. Place the forehead on the mat; look down the front of the body. Pull the shoulders down from your ears and squeeze the shoulder blades together. Tighten the seat muscles.

Slowly start raising your head, skimming the forehead, nose, and chin forward on the mat.

Raise the chin. Feel the stretch across the throat. Feel the back of the head press lightly against the shoulder muscles.

Pull the shoulders down and back once again. (If the shoulders won't lower, adjust by sliding hands back a half inch.)

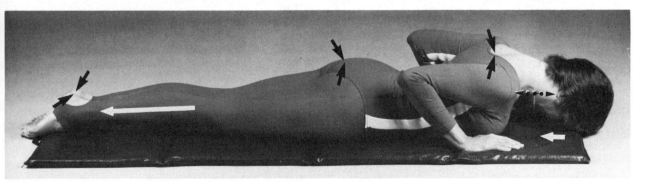

Cobra (beginning)

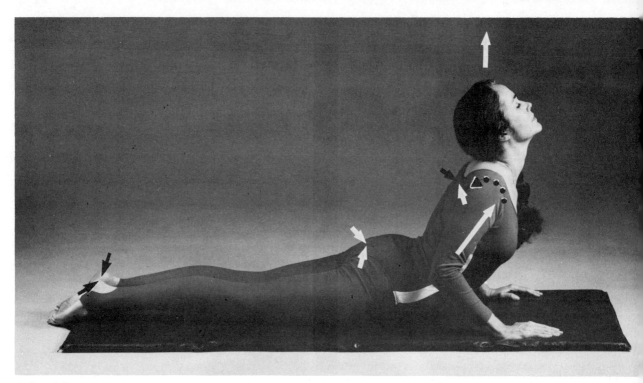

Cobra (lifting sternum)

Extend your legs back. Feet together.

Slowly arch the upper back until your navel *just* starts to come off the floor. Increase the shoulder squeeze. Then hold, breathing comfortably. Tilt the pelvis *firmly!*

Visualize your spine as you slowly lift up the sternum. Visualize each vertebra of the upper back as it becomes involved one by one; breathing is slow and relaxed. Use the hands to balance and to keep pressure on the entire spine, and close to the body. Elbows are bent. Hold top of the pose for 10 seconds, working up to 20. Breathe normally.

The descent is carried out with the same care as the ascent, with the back muscles controlling the descent as you maintain the shoulder squeeze and lead with the sternum. Keep the head back until the very end, then tuck in your chin, nose, and forehead; release the posture. Relax. Turn your head to the side and observe the sensations of the spine and back.

The entire pose should take about 15 seconds up to the top and 15 seconds down.

A breath I find extremely helpful and fun to do when doing the Cobra is the Pump Breath. I literally pump my chest off the ground with 8 or 10 little breaths. A "little" means inhaling the lung one-fourth full. It's very much like pumping up a flat tire or balloon.

As you lift each individual part of your body off the mat, use a separate little breath. For example:

Inhale, Pump Breath, lift chin, nose, and forehead. Exhale and hold head position. Inhale, Pump Breath, lift collarbone. Exhale, hold body position. Inhale, Pump Breath, lift breastbone. Exhale, hold body position. Inhale, Pump Breath, lift shoulders, hold. Exhale, hold, and so on.

On each hold, you maintain body position and height. Let your breath carry you up! Use very little hand pressure. Then once you're at "the top" take 5 breaths in and out of your navel, pretending the navel is a nostril and you are bringing in energy through your navel. Them pump yourself slowly down and relax.

Helpful Hints

Look down the front of your body to lengthen the neck.

Do the "skimming of the nose, etc., over the mat" with awareness. It is in this motion that you are contacting and directly stimulating the seven cervical vertebrae.

Remember to keep the shoulder blades squeezed during the movement.

Keep your legs together, or at least, hip distance apart.

Keep the buttocks muscles tightened throughout.

Tilt the pelvis at the top of the Cobra to prevent lower-back compression.

houlders up under the ears.
any position.

ve directions. Go to the top
nd hips to mat. Inhale. Tilt

our right shoulder.
ead to center.
...ad look over your left shoulder.
Inhale and bring head to center.
Exhale and slowly descend to the mat.

Cobra Variation 2

Lie on the mat. Hands are in line with the breast-bone.

Proceed with the Cobra. At the top of the Cobra straighten the elbows, rotate the "eyes" inside of your elbows to face forward. Tilt the pelvis firmly; lift the hips and knees 3 inches off the mat. Toes flat. Pull the kneecaps up.

Pull the shoulders down from the ears and squeeze the shoulders together.

Release. Bend the elbows and bring your hips to the floor. Slowly descend to the mat.

Cobra Variation 3

Do the regular Cobra. Take 1 minute to go up and 1 minute to go down, counting *om-1, om-2, om-3,* etc.

Helpful Hints

Do the Pelvic Tilt with real firmness. It takes the pressure off the lower back.

COBRA SALUTE

Varying the pose keeps the posture fresh and interesting, firms the upper arms, and increases spinal flexibility.

Lie down on the mat. Your face is to the mat. Place the right hand, palm down, directly beneath your face, nose to your knuckles. The left arm is pressed against the left ear, hand extended out as far as possible. Heels of your feet together. (See photo.)

Inhale; then exhaling, come up onto the right elbow, lifting the left arm up, keeping it close to your ear. (See photo.)

Inhale; then press down firmly onto the palm of your right hand. Straighten the elbow, keeping the elbow close to your rib cage. At the top of the pose, pull the right shoulder down from your ear!

Inhale, elongate your spine, and extend the line

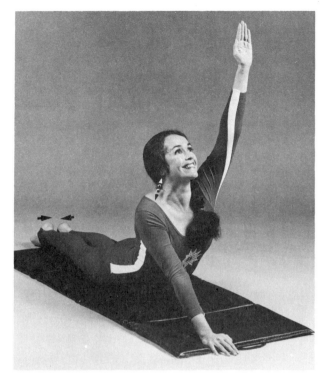

Cobra Salute

of the navel to the sternum. Exhale, lift your eyes toward the fingertips, and salute higher. Tilt your pelvis.

Inhale; then, exhaling, come down slowly, extend your sternum forward, reaching out to the wall in front of you as you come down.

Make a pillow of your hands. Inhale; then exhaling, take a deep breath, resting with your feet way apart.

Bring the feet together and then repeat on opposite side.

Helpful Hints

If your wrists are weak, place the hand farther forward on the mat. Concentrate on elongation and pelvic tilt of your back, which will relieve some of the arm pressure.

FLYING LOCUST

This strengthens the muscles of your lower back and brings a fresh supply of blood to the brain and to the skin of the face. Keeps elbows flexible. A deep massage for the uterus.

Step 1

Lie with your chin on the mat. Make a fist with each hand. Lift your hips off the mat and slip the

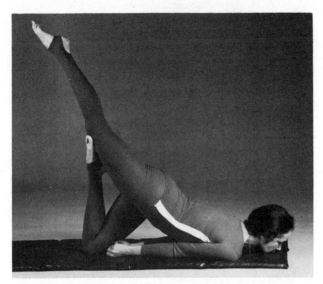

Flying Locust

arms beneath your torso. Thumbs and eyes, instead of your elbows, are on the mat. Your fists are together (note hands in photo).

Step 2

Draw your knees up to touch the fists.

Step 3

Exhale and tighten your right buttock. Lift the right leg, pointing the toes. Inhale, bend the left leg at the knee, and place the left foot over the right knee.

Exhale and relax in this lovely position. Come down and repeat Flying Locust on the other leg.

HALF LOCUST

Go through Steps 1 and 2 for the Flying Locust. Exhale, then raise the right leg up and extend your heel. Take another inhalation. Keep hips parallel to the floor. Exhale, push down on your fist, lower the leg, and repeat on the opposite side.

FULL LOCUST (SALABHASANA)

Repeat Steps 1 and 2 for the Flying Locust. Exhale. As you tighten the seat, push down on your arms and thrust both legs vigorously toward the ceiling.

Inhale once again. Exhale, arms to the mat. Slowly come down. Pull arms from under you. Relax and make a pillow of your hands. Feet wide apart. Take a deep breath. Bravo!

BOW (DHANURASANA)

The Sanskrit word for bow is Dhanus. This Bow is a little bit different from the classical posture found in traditional Yoga books. The object of this Bow is to keep as much compression as possible out of the lower back and to open the upper chest and the area in between the shoulder blades. It should be done on an empty bladder and with a firm mat. The arms are the sinew of the bow, the legs the shaft.

The Bow firms the abdomen, and it firms arms and bustline. Elasticity often lost through age, diet, and tensions may be returned to the entire spine. It is said to improve balance and memory.

Lie on your abdomen on your mat and place a firm blanket or pillow just below the abdomen. If needed, adjust your pillow to where it helps elevate you the highest. Place your chin on the mat. Grasp your ankles firmly, keeping the knees hip distance 12 inches apart. Arms are straight.

Inhale, looking down the front of your body. Exhale, and lift the forehead, nose, and chin. Now start to tighten buttocks and straighten your knees slightly, still holding on to the ankles. Feet flat. Inhale and squeeze the shoulder blades together and lift your breastbone high up toward the ceiling. Elongate and relax your neck. Exhale, release pose slightly. Then inhale, lifting your chest and rib cage off the floor, pulling your hands as leverage against the ankles. Your thighs must stay flat to the floor. Keep your neck free at all times.

Stay and hold in this Bow. Inhale and exhale. On each inhalation, release slightly; then on exhalation, lift the sternum even higher. Repeat 3 times; then remove pillow and relax.

Once you have worked with the pillow for a few weeks, remove it, and do entire pose without it.

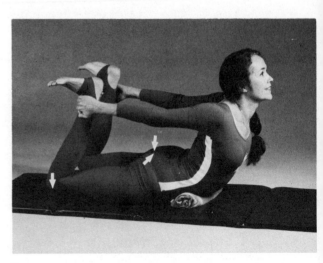

Bow

Lilias, Yoga, and Your Life

Variation

Try this hand variation to get deeply into that stubborn area between the shoulder blades.

Grab hold of the inside of your ankles, elbows straight (note photo), knees 12 inches apart. Now proceed with the entire Bow pose. Great!

SIDE BOW

The photo of the variation on the theme of the Bow pose gives you an opportunity to see the outer workings of the Asana posture from an aerial view. Notice that the heels of the feet are in line with the hips, thus giving a safe and comfortable stretch to the knees. The shoulder blades are squeezed together tightly. The ankles are pressed into your hands for leverage. Feet are flat or pointed.

This is also a nice way to do the Bow if you are pregnant—without the rolling, of course. (See chapter 17.)

Follow the procedure for the Bow (without a pillow).

Then slowly roll over onto the right side; look way over your left shoulder. Inhale and arch the spine; exhale and roll to the other side. Ease the arch as you roll.

To roll to the right, lift the left leg high; the rest of the body will follow. Rock from side to side 4 or 5 times.

For a stronger arch, press the knees and feet together when you are on your side.

Release, relax, and rest on your side.

Helpful Hints

When doing your Bow pose, if the pubic or hip bone feels tender due to lack of padding, by all means place an unfolded, firm blanket beneath your hips.

FULL SHOULDERSTAND

Consider your spinal column. It contains 24 cylindrical bones (vertebrae) stacked one on top of the other like spools of thread. These 24 vertebrae are amazingly strong and resilient, bearing 90 percent of your body weight.

The upper neck, called the cervical curve of your spine, contains seven vertebrae. Drop your chin to your chest; reach around and feel the protruding bones of your neck at the collar line. The largest protrusion felt at the nape of the neck is a cervical vertebra. (Note photo, next page.)

The neck becomes a bridge in the Shoulderstand.

The cartoid arteries run in conjunction with the internal jugular veins, vagus nerves, and muscles of the neck. In the Shoulderstand these arteries should be pumping blood freely down this bridge into the head. At the same time blood is pooling in and around the throat muscles and thyroid area.

It is vital that we Yoga students find the safest, most comfortable position of the neck and shoulders so as to keep this blood flowing freely through the bridge of the neck and into the brain during the Shoulderstand. We must also learn to protect the delicate neck vertebrae.

Picture yourself in the Shoulderstand and visualize, while in this inverted position, almost all your body weight resting totally on those delicate upper-neck vertebrae.

Year after year of pressure on the cervical curve of the neck from your own body weight will leave a rough callous or dark bruise, even start upper-neck soreness, stiffness, or more serious problems, in some cases where there were *none* to begin with!

Therefore, take a few precautionary measures.

1. Rotate your shoulders during the pose. See "Building Blocks," chapter 5, page 15.

The Shoulder Rotation is not too difficult to do in this upside-down position; yet, I have found that I can never rotate enough. The elbows always seem to slip out, and I slightly lose the rotation. I like doing the Shoulderstand wearing a T-shirt because I can use my hands against the skin of my back to keep me straighter.

2. Use one or two firm blankets beneath your shoulders for support.

To protect the upper neck, elevate the area with either your folded Yoga mat or one or two firm woolen blankets. The mat, plus the blanket that I'm using in this picture, is excellent because it is not wrinkly and forms a neat, clean line beneath my neck and shoulders. I also will occasionally use just wool blankets folded properly and neatly and placed precisely parallel to the shoulders. They are *not* meant to bunch up and look like an accordion beneath the neck (note photo), nor are they meant to support the back of your head. The blanket or a *good* firm Yoga mat is to be used to lift up and make a cushion on the vertebrae of the upper neck. I also feel rather strongly that *everyone*—teacher and student alike—should always do a Shoulderstand with this added support.

3. For complete freedom of your neck in the Shoulderstand remove all heavy necklaces. Also, never do Shoulderstand with hair bunched under the nape of your neck. Pull long hair or hair in a bun off to one side.

The Shoulderstand is one of the best possible

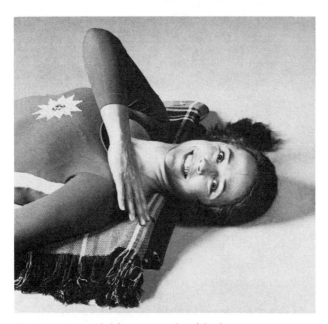

Correct way to fold your woolen blanket.

postures (Asanas). *Sarvangasana*, the Sanskrit name, comes from *sarv* (all) and *anga* (parts). Literally translated, it means "whole body posture"—perfectly named because this posture works on us from head to toe.

What a delicious tonic it is for the body to be turned upside down for a few minutes away from the pull of gravity that constantly tugs at veins, arteries, and organs.

This posture improves circulation to such important areas as the spine, the brain, the pelvic area. The thyroid gland is said to be stimulated in this posture, especially when this pose is released.

Asthma, throat ailments, and breathlessness are said to be affected positively because of increased circulation to the chest and neck.

This pose is supposed to be beneficial for menstrual cramps, hemorrhoids, and urinary disorders.

It relaxes and releases tensions throughout the whole body, thus aiding insomnia sufferers.

It gives new vitality and energy.

Fold your mat, or place a firm, folded blanket on the mat or floor, as shown in photo. Lie down and place the shoulders on the material to elevate the cervical vertebrae. Do not get material bunched up above the shoulders. With the arms alongside the body, palms down, contract your seat muscles and tilt the pelvis.

Inhale deeply; then exhaling, slowly raise both legs to a right angle; extend your heels toward the ceiling. Holding the legs in a right-angle position, inhale deeply; then, exhaling, push down on the hands and elbows and lift your hips from the floor. (Be sure this is done on the exhalation.) As the hips raise off the floor, immediately support the back with your hands and get your balance.

At this point, rotate your shoulders. (Clasp your hands together; straighten the elbows, and squeeze both shoulders in toward the spine.) If you lose your balance doing this rotating maneuver, bend the knees.

As you press the elbows into the mat, release your hands and support the back, trying to keep the elbows as close together as possible.

At this point, go through the following mental checklist:

1. Are the elbows and shoulders pressed to the floor?
2. Is there a comfortable space between the chest and chin?
3. Are the buttocks muscles tightened in a Pelvic Tilt?
4. Is the spine stretched straight upward?
5. Are the balls of the feet lifted toward the ceiling?

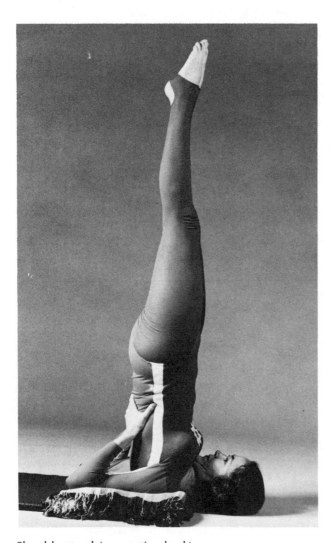

Shoulderstand (supporting back)

Lilias, Yoga, and Your Life

6. Are the nose, chin, and sternum in perfect alignment?
7. Are the hands moving downward toward the shoulder blades?

Hold this position for 1 to 5 minutes, breathing comfortably. (The abdominal muscle is often weak in the beginning, thus allowing the organs behind the abdominal wall to push downward on the lungs, causing shallow breathing. Continue with leg lifts and sit back, and soon this area will be strong and supportive.)

Come down, bringing knees to forehead, using your hands on the floor as a brake. Keeping your head on the floor, roll each vertebra to the floor, using the back and abdominal muscles.

Lie flat on your back; relax and observe how this posture has affected your legs, torso, arms, and face.

If a slight tightening occurs in the lower back after coming down, do a Pelvic Tilt or the rock-and-roll movement in chapter 7. This is due to the muscle weakness in the lower back and abdomen. It will disappear as the body gets stronger. Don't be concerned about it!

Helpful Hints

Place your hands beneath your shirt, directly onto the skin. Push against the skin to help you bring your hands higher.

Keep working upward while you are in the posture; do not sleep in it!

Tighten your buttocks and rear thighs; these are the muscles that keep you stretching up vertically.

Hold the posture for 1 to 2 minutes; then in a year's time, work up to 5 minutes.

Use your hands as brakes to return to the mat.

Keep a watch hung onto your tights or shorts to help you keep track of time.

Follow the Shoulderstand with the Fish.

Do not let the blanket bunch under your neck.

Do not lean into the neck. Work away from it.

Do not move your head while in the Shoulderstand.

The experienced student should come out of this pose with legs straight.

Variations on the Shoulderstand

After you have been holding the pose for 2 to 3 minutes and feel strong and confident, then proceed with the variations. They add spice and variety.

1. Legs in V position.
2. Inhale. Exhaling, lower the right toe to the floor behind your head. Left toe toward ceiling. Both knees remain straight. Return right leg

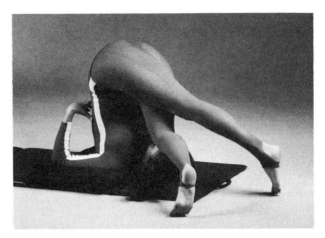

Variation 7

to vertical position. Repeat on the opposite leg.
3. Legs together and straight, turn your hips to the right, then the left.
4. Legs apart in a V, twist at the waist; legs are immobile in the hip joints.
5. Legs straight, heels together, toes out, keeping the turned-out extension. Then, legs apart in a V.
6. Legs straight, toes touching, heels out, legs apart in a V.
7. Inhale; then, exhaling, lower the right toe down to the floor behind your head. Let the right toe drift to the left. Cross the left leg over the right thigh. Both toes are on the floor. This is a scissors cross. Unwind slowly to keep your balance. Repeat on the opposite side.
8. Place your hands on the knees, legs remaining straight. Relax in the Pose of Tranquility. (See page 132.)

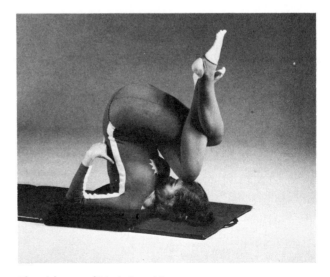

Shoulderstand Variation 10

Other Postures and Poses

9. Place your hands alongside the thighs. Think *body straight*. Balance on your shoulders.
10. Wrap your right thigh over the left thigh. Repeat in opposite direction.
11. Reach up and bring the right foot high onto the left thigh. Inhale; then exhaling, lower the right foot to the floor behind the head, knee straight. Release and change to the opposite leg.
12. Fold your legs, knees pointing toward the ceiling. Keep your spine straight and press the pelvis forward. Support the back. Hold for 30 seconds. Then release your back, place hands on knees, legs in balance.

FISH OVER A BARREL

Men and women who have excessively round shoulders, respiratory complaints such as asthma, or a tendency toward colds, have what I call a sleepy torso. It's as if there is no life in the chest or back area!

The Fish and all its variations bring energy, new circulation, and life force directly into these sleepy areas of muscle, nerves, lungs, heart and skin of the upper body.

Fish Over a Barrel is just a name for torso stretch, using the aid of a rolled-up blanket or small footstool. I suggest *everyone* do it, the advanced student as well as the beginner.

Beginners will get in touch with new areas of their upper body. Advanced students can make this stretch more difficult, thereby improving the muscle stretch for later postures such as the Wheel and Scorpion.

Take about 4 firm, not bouncy blankets, wool if possible, and fold them in thirds.

Roll one blanket over another until you have a nice 3-foot-high blanket roll. This roll must be soft but solid. (For these photos I am using a curved footstool with a folded blanket. Either a firm blanket roll or footstool with a blanket will work beautifully.)

Place the small of your back a few inches away from the blanket roll or stool. Then lean against the roll with the arms at your sides, and arch the spine over and back. Take 3 or more deep breaths, letting your head drop back comfortably.

After your chest and back muscles have stretched out, raise the arms up toward the ceiling and back over your head, close to the floor. Relax the muscles in your shoulders and armpits. Take 3 deep breaths.

If you are excessively stiff, holding the arms in this position can be extremely uncomfortable. If so, omit. To come out of the stretch, if you have a weak upper neck, place one hand behind the curve of the upper neck for support, and then raise your head up.

Helpful Hints

For more added stretch, place two cans of soup in either hand for added weight as you add arm lifts.

Adjust the lower-back position if you feel pain.

Do not force.

BEGINNER'S FISH (MATSYASANA)

Matsya in Sanskrit means fish. This posture is supposed to resemble a fish leaping out of water. The Fish should always follow the full Shoulderstand position. In the Shoulderstand, the blood pools around the thyroid area of the neck. In the Fish position, this area of the throat is opened and stretched in the opposite direction. This stimulation of the thyroid area with fresh blood is said to im-

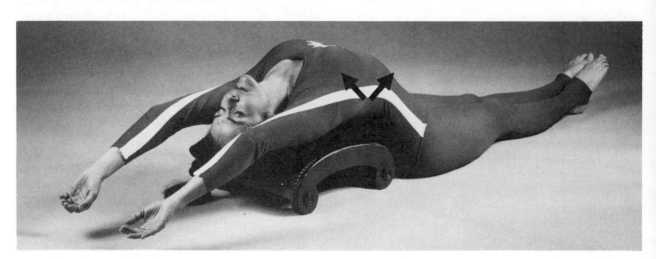

Fish Over a Barrel (footstool)

prove the metabolism of the body. Perhaps this is why students often say they lose extra pounds slowly and normally, or gain weight with more ease, if a few pounds are needed.

This posture is tremendously helpful for men, women, and children suffering from asthma and shortness of breath. The chest is fully expanded, thus improving breathing and lung circulation. The nerves in the upper back and neck are affected by this pose. I suggest you read "Back Talk," chapter 13.

If you feel slightly nauseated after doing the Fish, don't feel discouraged. This feeling of vertigo will pass with time and practice.

Lie on your back.

Place your hands under the seat muscles, palms down, fingers pointing forward. Be sure you are *sitting on your hands and wrists* all during the posture. (Note photo.)

Inhaling, arch your spine and lift your entire back off the floor. Roll the head back and rest the crown of your head lightly on the floor.

Think *sternum (breastbone)* up. Squeeze the shoulder blades together.

The weight of this posture rests on the elbows, not on the top of your head.

Inhale deeply. Exhale and inhale completely, twice.

Then, inhaling, come out of the posture. Exhale, release your hands, and relax.

FISH (MATSYA)

Lie on your back; bend the knees and cross your ankles; hold onto instep, right hand to left instep, left hand to right instep.

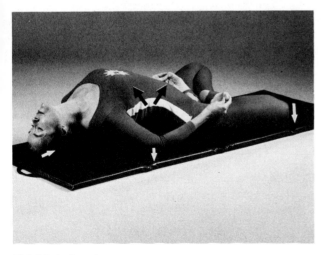

Fish Variation 1

Place your feet and knees on the mat.

Press your elbows firmly into the mat.

Inhale and arch the spine, lifting the sternum toward the ceiling. Exhale and arch the neck, rolling your head back until the crown touches the mat.

Breath deeply several times.

Remember, the weight is on your elbows, buttocks, crossed ankles, and the crown of your head (lightly); squeeze shoulders together.

Release after holding 5 to 30 seconds.

Variation 1

Lie down on the mat with the aid of your elbows.

Inhale. Arch the spine and squeeze shoulders, lift the sternum and roll back on your head. Exhale. Work your knees closer to your mat, reaching for your toes.

Hold 10 to 60 seconds, breathing deeply.

Inhale and relax. Repeat with legs crossed in the opposite direction.

Variation 2

Sit on your knees. Temporarily you can have the knees farther apart than hip distance. However, the goal is to gradually have the knees touch.

Lower the weight to your elbows. If the knees come off the ground at this point, do *not* proceed! As your thigh muscles stretch out, the rest of this movement will become possible.

Lower yourself to your elbows; lift the sternum; arch the spine; roll back lightly to the crown of the head. Use the leverage from your hands holding your ankles to maintain shoulder squeeze. Bring the knees together as the thigh muscles become more comfortable. Hold for 3 to 5 complete breaths. With each breath open the chest and continue shoulder squeeze.

Then to return to Step 1, firmly clasp your ankles, squeeze the shoulder blades together, and raise the head. Press the elbows into the floor and come up onto the elbows. Sliding your hands down toward your toes, go 2 inches beyond your toes. Place weight evenly on both hands and sit up without twisting.

Variation 3

When in the Fish position you can move your hands to a prayer position over the chest.

Or, as you continue to stretch the arched chest up toward the ceiling, bring the hands back over your head to touch the mat. For a third hand position, inhale and place fingers behind the neck, thumbs across your throat. Elbows touch the mat. Inhale deeply.

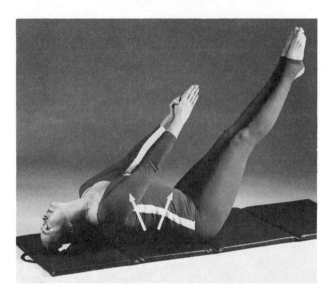

Fish Variation 4

These might be a strain for problem necks, so caution is advised.

Variation 4

Go to top of the Fish with your legs straight (Beginner's Fish).

Inhale and raise the arms toward the ceiling, palms together. Exhale and lower your arms.

Variation 5

Go to top of the Beginner's Fish pose. Raise both arms toward ceiling.

Exhaling, tilt the pelvis and raise the legs up to the ceiling.

Inhale again as you reinforce the lift.

Helpful Hints

Remember to breath smoothly and deeply in the pose.

Have the crown of your head lightly touching the floor, weight on the buttocks. *No strain on the neck!*

Do not get discouraged if you feel slightly nauseated on the first tries of the Fish. Just come out of the pose and take 3 Complete Breaths. This vertigo should pass quickly as your body gets used to the Asana.

HEADSTAND PUSHUP (DOLPHIN)

This promotes confidence in the headstand and develops control, coordination, and strength.

Read instructions thoroughly before trying the exercise.

Sit on your knees. Lean forward and place your elbows on the mat. Measure the distance between your elbows by placing your left fist against your right elbow. (Note photos.)

Clasp your hands together with the heels of your hands touching, thumbs crossed. Your little fingers are pressed together. Place the crown of your head on your mat. (Note to experienced students: This hand position I have found to be very comfortable because it shifts the weight around. It feels a little strange in the beginning, but I like it! It keeps my upper neck straight and is very relaxing for my hands. If you find it is not for you, go back to the old way of hands cupped around your head, thumbs up, but do give this method a try.)

Straighten your knees and curl your toes under.

Turn your wrists inward. Press your upper arm down and your forearms into the mat. This will give you leverage to lift your head off the mat.

Inhale, exhale, pushing in on your wrists and down on your upper elbows. Lift your head up and down a few inches off the mat. Keep looking at your toes. Lean back, lifting your shoulders up and back, shoulder blades together.

Relax; then repeat 4 times.

Release, bend your knees, keep your elbows on the mat. To check to see if your elbows drifted farther apart, remeasure.

Traveling elbows are a sign of weak upper arms.

After you feel comfortable with this pushup, walk your toes in toward your face until you feel more weight on your elbows; then repeat the above process, lifting 4 times. Relax and repeat.

Helpful Hints

Do not do this or any exercise half on your mat and half off.

Do not grip with your hands. Pushing down on your forearms will give you leverage.

Keep your knees straight.

HEADSTAND (SIRSHASANA)

I have always been a traditionalist so far as doing the Headstand without the use of a wall. Preparing the body and mind to be as strong as a wall has always made sense to me. However, visions of men and women collapsing in their living rooms while watching the TV Yoga class might have something to do with my having changed my mind about using a wall.

Please read the following steps carefully. Visualize yourself going through all the different stages. Then imagine yourself going through the motions of the Headstand without the wall and then possibly losing your balance. How would you handle it? Would you be fearful and freeze, or would you round your back and roll over easily and with control, tucking your chin toward your throat, relaxing your body? You need time for this pose. Be the explorer. Take one step at a time. If you have questions about high blood pressure or neck problems, please consult your family doctor. By the way, when I refer to "the crown" of the head, it means that exact point where the 4 sides of your skull meet at the top of your head.

Because of the reversal of the normal upright position, the following are benefits derived from the Headstand:

Circulation to your brain is greatly improved as well as to the eyes, ears, and heart. The nervous system is toned. Your abdominal organs that can normally sag or prolapse, are pulled into proper position. Sinus fluids are permitted a downward flow. Constipation problems are generally improved. Colds, sore throats, insomnia, "nerves," headaches, asthma, and varicose veins are supposed to be improved!

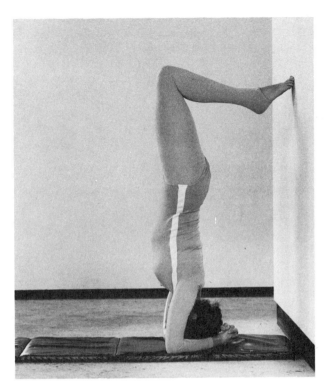

Headstand (Step 2)

Step 1

Kneel on the floor, knees close together. Measure the distance between your elbows. Place your palms together, fingertips to the wall. Interlace fingers, thumbs crossed, heels of hands pressed together. Your hand is about 5 inches from the wall.

Place the crown of your head on the mat and fit the back of your head in the V of your wrists. Your eyebrows should be parallel to the floor. Recheck to see that your knees are in line with your elbows.

Tuck your toes under and straighten your legs; tailbone up toward the ceiling. Place the weight on your forearms and elbows by leaning back. Your spine will be straight as you tilt back *just enough* to note that your knees automatically want to bend toward your body and your feet come off the floor. Bring one knee at a time to your chest and *hold*. *Do not kick up*. Get used to feeling upside down. Should you lose your balance in Step 1, it is very easy to recover and start again.

Step 2

Press down and use the strength in your forearms and elbows. Raise both knees. Bring your feet above your spine. Touch the toes of both feet lightly to the wall. (Heels will cause you to lose balance.) With your toes lightly touching the wall, straighten and adjust your shoulders and head position, if needed. Maintain your controlled Headstand, Step 2, from this position. The spine is straight. Hold, breathing

shallowly. Only after you can hold Step 2 with confidence and no shakiness, should you proceed to Step 3.

Step 3

Without moving the body from hips down, slowly raise both feet up directly above the spine, about 3 inches from the wall. When the knees are straight and you feel more confident, check to see that you are not arching your spine. If you are, correct this by pulling your rib cage in, then your legs apart slightly, contracting the buttocks muscles and tipping the pelvis. Then bring your legs together again, *holding* this solid feeling in the lower back.

Hold this pose for 30 seconds. Time yourself. (Place a clock in front of you.) Add on a few seconds every other day. Work up to 3 to 10 minutes.

Reverse the pattern used to go up in order to come down. Rest in Pose of a Child (see page 92). Never bounce up quickly after this Asana.

Helpful Hints

Use the wall at first if it gives you confidence. Then after a few weeks, move your practice to the center of the room.

Move your hands slightly away from the wall if the contour of your seat prevents you from getting proper wall alignment.

Remember to breathe during the posture.

Other Postures and Poses

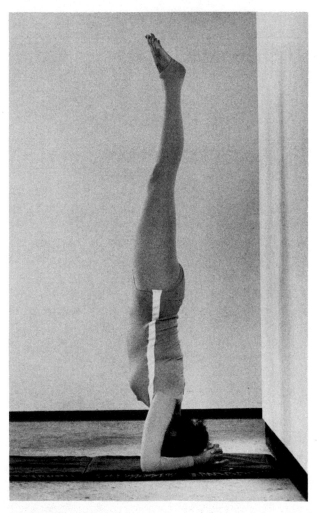

Headstand (Step 3)

Relax your face and neck, keeping eyebrows parallel to the floor.

Remove your finger rings when doing the Headstand. This prevents undue stress on fingers and joints. (Remember to put them back on immediately when through.)

Recheck your elbows after the Headstand. See if your elbows have moved!

Practice the Headstand after warmups and at the beginning of your daily practice when you are fresh and strong.

Let the Headstand follow the Shoulderstand.

Be patient and take your time. Soon the pieces of this puzzle will fit together.

Variations

These are to be attempted when you are comfortable and confident and *do not* need the reassurance of the wall. Then have some fun with these variations.

Follow Steps 1–3. Then:

1. Spread your legs apart in a V.
2. Inhale, exhale and lower right leg to the mat behind your head. (Bend at the waist.) Inhale up. Repeat with the opposite leg. Repeat three times each leg.
3. Inhale, exhale and lower both legs to the mat behind your head. (Lean back slightly as you lower, maintaining control.) Go as far as you can; then return. Soon your toes will lightly touch the mat. Don't rest them there. Use your abdominal muscles. Keep your legs straight throughout the pose.
4. Spread your legs and twist from your hips, legs immobile at the joints.
5. Cross your thighs. Spread your legs apart from this position.
6. Inhale, placing your right foot inside your left thigh. Exhale, lowering your left leg to the mat. Repeat on the opposite leg.
7. With soles of feet together, bring your knees sideways in a straight line to the body.
8. Bend both knees, letting your legs hang loosely back behind you. With back arched and chest pressed forward, tighten your seat and tip your pelvis.
9. Place the right foot on the left knee. Reverse the position.

Helpful Hints

Do not slump into your shoulders. Remind yourself to constantly create space between the shoulder area and the ears.

Keep the wrists straight.

Do not roll wrists inward.

Use these variations to keep your practice fresh and fun.

FORWARD BEND (PASCHIMOTTANASANA)

If you get stuck in your Forward Bend poses, the chances are that the back of your legs, as well as your stiff spine and hips, is the culprit. Take your time and be patient with these stubborn areas. Faithfully work with stepping-stone leg stretches with a tie. Use a telephone book beneath your sitting bones (as in photo) if you are very stiff. It cants you forward very naturally. I know this is an uncomfortable pose when you first start. But keep persevering! In three months you'll be *much* closer and feel less discomfort. I couldn't do it either 15 years ago.

Also, remember to try and get as much muscle and skin from the back of the thighs on the mat as possible *before* you go forward. When you simply *sit* on those muscles, you squeeze off their capacity for more stretch. All I do to achieve this maneuver is to rock over to my right thigh; then I pull over to the left and pull the right muscle out.

How to Work with Excessive Stiffness in Forward Bend

Place a solid, thick book (telephone directory or dictionary), or folded blanket beneath your sitting bones (ishium). You will be elevated approximately 2 inches off the ground. This elevation will eliminate much of the muscle discomfort of a forward bend. The lift also encourages your spine to lean forward naturally and effortlessly.

Now, place a soft tie or belt under the balls of your feet. As you firmly hold onto the tie, try flattening your feet and pressing the backs of the knees to the floor.

Next, hold firmly (midthigh) onto the belt. Slowly, with no bouncing, pull your upper body forward about 3 inches, concentrating on the rotation-of-the-hip motion, keeping the feet flat and legs straight. Do not force or give in to the rounded spine. Elongate the spine. Lead from the sternum. Hold this position 30 seconds to one minute. Breathing shallowly, talk to the muscles holding you back. Suggest to them that they relax, especially as you exhale.

Inhale; then sit up once again. Sit tall. Repeat the above. Exhale; keep leading with the sternum. Hips are still rotating. Shoulder blades are pulled down and back.

Work your elbows back and close to the body.

Take 3 to 5 deep breaths within the hold of the posture.

Release and relax.

Our demonstrator is Diana Noyes, member of the Cincinnati Yoga Teachers Association.

Diana shows us how using the tie properly will aid the rotation of the hips, the elongation of the spine, and the leading and lifting from the sternum. With each inhalation, she pulls on the tie, which gives her leverage to rotate her hips and moves her lower spine into a concave position. With each exhalation, her sternum is kept high. Note the tie is under the balls of her feet.

Remember, it's not how low you go, but how you get there!

One of the basic principles of why Yoga works is the simple squeeze-hold-release that happens within the body as you do the poses. In the Forward Bend,

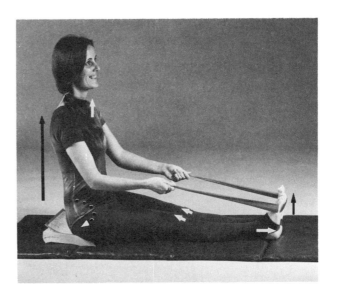

Forward Bend (with tie)

the muscles that hold the vital organs of the body in place are compressed. This means of course, that the stomach, liver, spleen, kidneys, pancreas, colon and intestines are being squeezed or are gently massaged as you hold the forward position. Then as you release, a fresh supply of blood rushes into these organs, cleaning, removing toxins, and nourishing with blood.

Sit on the mat, feet together. Reach down and pull out the back side of your thigh muscles to touch as much of the mat as possible.

Raise the arms above your head. Inhale, stretching upward, sitting tall. The head stays between the upper arms; spine is straight.

Inhale and raise the arms up toward the ceiling. Lift up and out of your hips. Feel as if you are putting space between each rib.

Smoothly exhaling, extend the body forward only 2 inches. Rotate your hips; lift the chin, but keep the neck relaxed and the spine elongated.

Inhale and now extend the body forward 4 inches. Hold and place your hands on the ankles, or catch the toes. (Hold the toes with your thumbs and first two fingers.) Kneecaps are pulled up. No light beneath the knees, please!

Continue the forward motion, always leading with the breastbone, neck free from tension. Toes are pulled back, foot flattened. Your elbows rest on the floor.

Draw abdomen muscles upward to extend the forward bend. For the first three months, *forget* about bringing your head to your knees.

Hold for 30 seconds, working up to 5 minutes.

As you hold, work your breathing into this

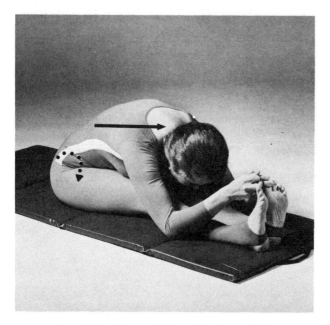

Forward Bend (leading with breastbone, neck free)

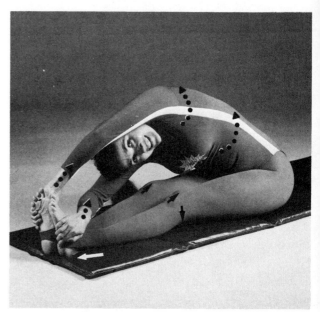

Forward Bend (twist position)

stretch, playing the edges of your forward bend. (Inhale, pull back, relaxing slightly; then exhale and come forward to where you begin to feel the aliveness of your legs and hips.) It is a "sweet" sort of discomfort but no pain! Think *hold a little behind my maximum edge*, talking to the muscles and ligaments that hold you back.

When your chest fully reaches the thighs, then lower your head toward the knees. This takes many months of work, so please don't force this pose!

To release, inhale and stretch the body upward, raising your arms slowly; reach toward the ceiling. Exhale. Return to your mat; bend the knees; feet are flat. Round the spine and return the spine to the floor, one vertebra at a time.

Relax. Observe how the entire body feels!

Variation 1

Several hand positions are possible. You may clasp the fingers around the soles of the feet, or clasp the soles of the feet by bringing the wrists over the toes. Hold feet flat in this position.

Variation 2

Sit tall, legs straight out, feet together. Pull out the back of the thighs.

Raise your arms above the head and cross them, left over right, thumbs toward the floor.

Exhale and bend forward and clasp outer soles of each foot. Arms are still crossed. Breathe normally.

Inhale. Exhale and bend the elbows; twist the upper body to the right by pulling against your right

foot with your left hand, bringing your head between the arms. Look up.

Hold the pose for 5 to 30 seconds. Work with your breathing within the pose, twisting, trying to bring your navel toward the center of the pose, and exhaling simultaneously.

Inhale, release arms, sit tall. Exhale.

Repeat, reversing the arms and twisting to the left.

Helpful Hint

Pull against the right foot with the left hand. This will act as a lever to give you a deeper twist.

Variation 3

I really love to do the Forward Bend from this inverted position. It does take limberness. Once the pieces of this pose fit together you will feel a terrific release of tension and tightness in the lower back.

This exercise firms the thighs, increases back and hip flexibility, relieves lower-back pain, and promotes balance and self-confidence. And it feels wonderful!

Lie on your back on the mat. Legs are straight, arms are above the head, with the back of your hands on the floor.

Take a deep Complete Breath.

Inhale; then, exhaling, tilt the pelvis; slowly and smoothly raise the legs up toward the ceiling.

Clasp your hands around the ankles. Legs are straight, and kneecaps are pulled up. Your entire back is pressed to the floor.

Inhale; then exhaling, gently lift your lower back

Lilias, Yoga, and Your Life

off the mat by pulling your legs toward your face. By your applying pressure to ankles, elbows are out away from your body; lift your head slightly to meet the knees. (Note photo.) Release your lower back to the mat. Inhale and repeat, exhaling as your lower back lifts off the floor. Keep your knees straight throughout the exercise.

Do this pull-release motion 4 to 8 times.

Release your feet. Bring the knees to the chest, lower back to the floor. Then straighten your legs up toward the ceiling. On your exhalation, lower the legs to the floor. Relax and observe.

Helpful Hints

Try to bring your straightened knees to your face.

Keep the sacral and lumbar arch as close to the floor as possible throughout the exercise.

Relax the lower back when it is lifted off the floor.

Pull the kneecaps up.

10

More Postures and Poses

PLOW (HALASANA)

One must work up slowly to doing the Plow. It is a difficult posture to execute properly, especially when the back muscles are shortened and the spine is stiff. Warm up well for the Plow.

Using the chair in the Plow is just a modernization of this ancient exercise. Fifteen years ago a rounded spine would have been perfectly acceptable in class. Now, we are working toward a straighter spine, rotated hips, spinal safety within postures, and learning to hold for longer periods.

The Plow tones and pools blood around the thyroid and para-thyroid glands. It gives a complete stretch to the spinal cord, and the nerves and muscles of the legs. It is said to aid hypertension, constipation, muscular rheumatism and lumbago.

In Sanskrit *Hala* means plow because it resembles the very primitive plow of India. Read all the directions carefully before attempting this pose. Visualize yourself doing this posture perfectly. Then proceed cautiously and slowly into the Plow.

Lie down on your back with the legs straight, knees together; arms should be alongside the body.

Exhaling, do the Pelvic Tilt.

Inhale; then exhaling raise the legs to a vertical position, feet flat toward the ceiling. Keep the small of the back pressed to the mat.

Inhale; exhaling, pushing down on your hands, contract the abdominal muscles, and lift the hips. Draw your thighs close to the chest. This will aid in lifting the lower back off the floor.

Extend the legs over your head, lowering the toes to the mat. Do not force this.

Tighten the kneecaps. Rest for a moment.

Clasp your hands together behind you. Keep your arms on the mat. Straighten your elbows and rotate your shoulder blades in toward your spine.

Inhale, lifting up your hips and perineum (crotch) toward the ceiling.

Exhale and elongate the spine. The sixth and seventh cervical vertebrae of the spine should be recessed and completely off the mat.

Now release the hands and place them above your head.

Open your eyes and look into the hollow of the abdominal area. Rotate your hips by bringing the hip bones into and toward the upper-thigh muscles. This movement straightens the trunk of the body to form an approximate 90-degree angle.

Tighten the back of the thighs.

Hold the position for 1 minute, gradually working up to 5 minutes (after a few months).

Keep working while in the pose.

To come down, inhale, lower the arms, and press the palms of the hands firmly into the mat, keeping the legs straight, kneecaps raised, heels extended. Start lowering from the shoulder area. And press each vertebra to the floor. Keep the chin up and the back of the head to the floor; feel each vertebra as it touches the floor. Exhale slowly as you come down in a slow, controlled manner.

A more advanced way to come down is to raise the arms over the head, keeping the knees as close to your face as possible, legs straight. Slowly roll down, really stretching and lengthening your body

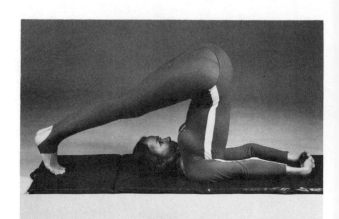

Full Plow (clasp hands behind you)

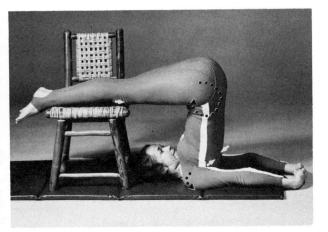

Plow with a Chair (rotating shoulder blades in toward spine)

all the way down. Inhale until hips touch the mat; then exhale and lower legs to the floor.

Helpful Hints

Never come crashing down in a lump after the posture is through.

If you collapse your chest in this posture, it puts undue pressure on your neck and chest and lungs. So keep working with the breathing rhythm. Inhale, extend; lift and elongate. Exhale and concave the back and tailbone toward the ceiling.

Now, go into the Plow and then do the following variations. Remember to rotate your shoulders.

Variation 1

Arms above your head on the mat, palms toward ceiling.

Bend both knees and bring knees on either side of your ears.

Try to touch your knees to the mat.

Feet remain together.

The special benefit of this variation is that the legs and the heart rest in this pose.

Variation 2

Spread the legs as far as possible, toes on the floor. Put your hands together and rotate the shoulders.

The special benefit of this variation is that it tones the legs and contracts the abdominal organs.

Variation 3

Go into the Plow.

Rotate your shoulders.

Release your hands; support the spine. Make your back as straight as possible.

Walk both feet as far as possible to the right, toes to the mat, knees straight.

Hold for 10 seconds.

Exhale, moving legs to the left. Hold for 10 seconds.

PLOW WITH A CHAIR

Find a good steady chair with no arms.

Place the chair approximately 12 inches behind your head. Turn the back of the chair sideways. (Note photo.)

Place the hands on the floor along the side of the body. Inhale; then, exhaling, lift both legs. Inhale; then exhale as your hips lift off the ground, using the arms to help you up. Place your lower legs comfortably on the seat of the chair. (Do not hang onto the chair as you go up.)

At this point, make the upper neck and shoulder area comfortable by rotating the shoulder blades in toward the spine and pulling shoulders down from ears. Arms are straight and on the mat. (Note photo.)

Open your eyes and look at your hip area. Remember the hip rotation you did while standing? Do the same thing now. Inhale, as if you are trying to bring the perineum (crotch) toward the ceiling; then exhale, bringing the hip bones in a circular motion toward your thigh muscles. You see? It's easy! Your spinal column is immediately straighter, and your cervical spine should be recessed and completely off the mat.

Now place the hands on your back as high as possible toward the shoulder blades.

The hand-to-back grip is firm; if you can, use the bare skin of your back. Fingertips are up toward the shoulders. Elbows are as close as possible to each other.

Holding this position, elongate the spine as you inhale. Then, concave, and rotate your hips extending the perineum again toward the ceiling as you exhale. There should be a comfortable space between your neck and chin. Breathing should be comfortable.

Repeat the breathing rhythm and practice with a chair until you understand the pose thoroughly. Repeat the movement 3 times. Then rest.

CROCODILE TWIST

This is an excellent spinal twist to release tension and tiredness in your lower back or to help realign spinal vertebrae. This simple twist can be accomplished after the spine is moderately free from constriction.

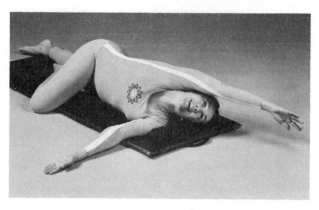

Crocodile

The hand and arm movements represent the jaws of the crocodile opening and closing; hence its name.

Lie on your back; bend the knees and place feet flat on the floor, about 12 inches away from the seat. Place the right foot on the left thigh.

Keep the foot on top of the thigh as you turn onto your left side. The bent right knee is now resting comfortably on the mat.

You are resting on your left shoulder. With arms outstretched, place palms of the hands together.

Look toward the thumb of your right hand. The arms symbolize the opening jaws of a crocodile. Watch the movement as you slowly raise your right arm and, skimming the floor by a few inches, reach toward the wall behind you and continue until your right arm forms a T position with the left arm, which has remained stationary.

When the arms reach a T position, press the shoulder blades into the floor; at this point your right knee will come off the floor. This is fine! Just relax the entire leg and breathe comfortably as you rest in the intensity of the stretch. Take 30 seconds to do this first movement.

As you hold this posture, tell yourself to relax the chest and upper arms, hips, and thighs.

Now place your left hand atop your right knee and gently press the knee a quarter inch toward the floor.

Attentiveness to breathing in this posture is important. On the inhalation, stretch and reach toward the walls of the room with your arms in a T. On the exhalation, gently press the knee to the floor.

When the knee and shoulders are easily on the floor, bring the arms back into the T pose. Work consciously with your breathing. On inhalation focus on stretching the arms and chest; on the exhalation stretch the lower back and leg.

Slowly release the posture in the same way you went into it. Watch the thumb of the right hand as your arms stretch over the head, returning to the original position of the hands together.

Turn over and repeat on the opposite side; then lie on your back, straighten the legs, and observe the body.

The entire exercise should take 1 or 2 minutes to do.

Helpful Hints

Slow the movement way, way down.

Feel the stretch from the tips of your toes to the tops of your fingers.

DOG STRETCH (MUKHASANA)

A perfect warmup, the Dog Stretch is also a good cooling down for the athlete. This exercise stretches the Achilles tendon; tones the arms, wrists, hips, ankles, and thighs; improves circulation to the head and heart and strengthens abdominal muscles. It is also recommended for arthritic shoulders.

Step 1

Lie on your back with feet 12 inches apart. Hands are directly beneath the shoulders. Curl your toes under. Inhale and jackknife your hips up toward the ceiling. Lift up onto the balls of the feet and bend yur knees.

Exhale, pushing with the palms of your hands into the mat. Pull your shoulders down from your ears, squeezing the blades together. Inhale; then, exhaling, elongate your spine and remember to lengthen the line between the navel and the sternum. Think *tailbone up to the ceiling.*

Take 3 complete rhythmic breaths, gently elongating the lower spine and making it concave on the exhalation. Relax.

Step 2

Repeat Step 1. Inhale; then, exhaling, straighten your legs, pull the kneecaps up and gently lower your heels to the mat. Hold at the edge of your stretch.

Inhale, pushing against the heels of your hands. Exhale, increasing your shoulder squeeze, with shoulders down from the ears.

Inhaling, feel the stretch of your legs. Exhale, with heels farther into the mat. Take 3 deep breaths with the stretching movements of this pose. This entire pose should take 30 seconds; then work up to a 1-minute hold.

Helpful Hints

If you have trouble keeping your heels to the mat, place the heels against a wall. Keep the hips

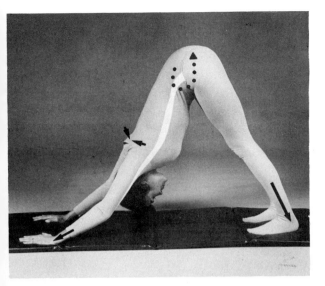

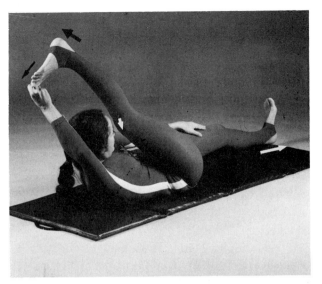

Dog Stretch (Step 2)   Spider

high and the arms straight. Keep working with your breath.

If you have difficulty in concaving your lower back, place the hands farther out in front of you.

Distribute your weight *evenly* over the heels of your hands and fingers. No white fingertips!

If you have bowed or extended elbows, do not lock them. Instead bend your elbows slightly; then bring them to a straight, but strong positioning.

Variation

Inhale, raising your right leg up and extending your heel; exhale, lowering your leg to the floor. Repeat 3 times on each leg.

SPIDER (SUPTA PADANGUSTHASANA)

This pose looks a little like a spider. Literally it means lying-down-foot-big-toe-pose. Quite a handle for such an intense stretch. This pose helps to relieve sciatica and gives a deep massage within the hip. It increases circulation and tones the entire leg.

As you lie on your back, legs are extended.

Place the left hand on your left leg. Bend the right knee, hugging it to your chest. Grab hold of the right big toe, wrapping your thumb and index finger around the toe. (Note photo.)

Inhale; then, exhaling slowly lift your head, simultaneously straightening the right knee. Then with the leg straight, bring your knee close to your nose. Extend the left heel intensely!

Hold for 5 to 20 seconds, breathing shallowly. Inhale. Lower the leg and repeat on the opposite side.

Helpful Hints

Before doing the spider, massage the back of both legs until they feel warm.

Keep the outstretched leg absolutely straight with heel on the floor.

It is more important to keep the right leg straight than to bring the knee to your nose.

Apply pressure from the left (thigh) hand around your right calf to help you come closer toward your face. Once you have stretched out, then return left hand to left thigh.

EAGLE

This tones your leg muscles, strengthens the ankles, and improves balance and stability.

Stand tall.

Balance on the left foot with the left leg bent. As you swing the right thigh around the front of the supporting left leg, continue wrapping the right foot; then lock your right foot around your left calf. Toes from the right foot point to the front, just above the inside of the left ankle.

As you cross the right elbow over the left elbow, clasp your hands together.

Slowly bend forward, lowering the elbows onto the knee. Chin is on the back of your hand.

Now extend the elbows outward, bending forward until the sternum rests on your bent upper thigh.

Hold the pose for 5 to 18 seconds, breathing rhythmically.

Slowly come up with the same control as you

More Postures and Poses   **67** went down into pose. Repeat on opposite leg, and cross left elbow over right.

Helpful Hints

Support yourself with a chair. If at first you lose your balance trying to wrap your legs remember to place your gaze 6 feet in front of you. Then as you bend forward, draw your gaze in to 3 feet. Try to keep your pose steady at the beginning, middle, and end.

FLYING BIRD (GARUD ASANA)

According to Hindu mythology, the *Garuda* was a magical bird of Lord Vishnu. It had the body of a bird and the head of a human. The *Garuda* was said to carry souls to heaven. One wing represented the grace of God; the other wing represented self-effort. Without both of these attributes, the soul would not be able to soar to the next plane.

The Flying Bird tones the entire body and increases stamina and concentration. And it's fun to do.

Stand off the mat, in a standing pose. Pull knee-caps up. Then gaze at a steady spot about 6 feet in front of you. Remember to draw the gaze in to 3 feet as you do this pose.

As you lift your left arm up toward the ceiling and keep the right arm to your side, extend the right leg behind you.

Inhale; then, as you exhale, extend the torso forward. The left arm is parallel to the floor and close to your left ear.

The right leg is now perfectly parallel to the floor. The right arm is straight alongside your body. (Feel as if you are trying to reach toward your right big toe with your right hand. You won't of course, but it should be that energized and straight.) This posture will appear like a bird in flight.

Repeat on opposite leg.

Hold for 30 seconds each side, breathing comfortably in the hold.

Do twice on each leg.

CAMEL

Using the wall increases your body awareness and the difficulty of the pose. This is an excellent stretch for back and thighs and neck. It's also good for ankle and foot flexibility.

Kneel and place the knees against a wall. Knees about 12 inches apart. Place your hands on the hips.

With the spine straight, tuck your pelvis, tightening the buttocks muscles. Lean back 4 inches, lifting up from the hips and ribs. Hold.

Now squeeze your shoulders firmly and lower your hands to touch your heels. (At first you may go one hand at a time, but for lower-back safety, lower both hands together as soon as possible.)

Inhaling, tighten your buttocks. Exhale and

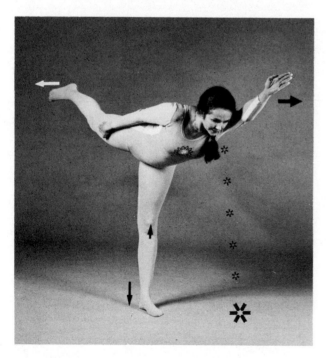

Garud Asana

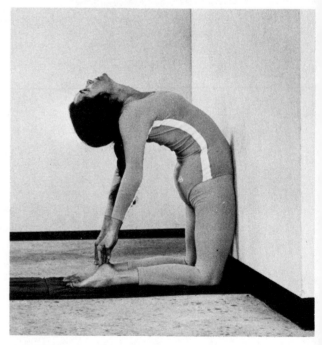

Camel

Lilias, Yoga, and Your Life

press your thighs forward to touch the wall. Repeat this breath and movement 2 more times.

Release both of your hands at exactly the same time. Lead with the navel, lift your chest and come up against the wall; then straighten your head.

FROG

Believe it or not, this is a very good exercise for tired legs, and, as the saying goes, "It feels great when you stop!"

Lying on your abdomen, feet 12 inches apart, rest the left cheek on your left hand. As you bend the right leg, reach back with the right hand, placing your toes at your wrists and grasping the instep.

Inhale; then pull the right shoulder blade in, back, and down from the ear. Your right elbow is high as you push the right heel down to touch your buttocks. Keep both hips to the mat. Play with this movement, using the rhythm of your breathing, until the heel touches your seat comfortably. Then continue.

Come up onto your left elbow, pushing the left hand down on the mat.

Turn and *look* at your right foot. Now *pivot* on the heel of the right hand and clasp your fingers over the toes. The right elbow is high.

Inhale and exhale, lift sternum and press heel to buttocks. Take 3 breaths to do this movement. Never, *never* force this movement.

After you have warmed up each foot, you will now lower both heels to your buttocks, using the above process. Keep your forehead to the mat, lifting the elbows. Do not force!

Release and come up to your knees.

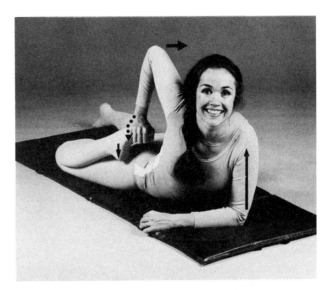

Frog (look at right foot)

FLOUNDER

This is rather difficult, and careful attention must be paid to your thighs, groin, abdomen, and to the warmups.

The Flounder tones up the entire spinal region firming the upper thighs and buttocks. Also increases stamina and confidence.

Kneel on the mat, with knees hip-distance apart. Then sit between your heels. Heels are turned outward, and your toes are close to your thighs, forming a slight curve.

Step 1

Carefully lean back and bring your weight to your elbows and rest there for a minute. Take two deep Complete Breaths and suggest to your knees and thighs to relax and stretch out. Open the knees farther if your knees are off the ground, or if there is any pain. Rest for 15 to 30 seconds in this position, letting the thighs stretch out gradually.

Step 2

Continue only if your knees are on the floor comfortably! Then lower the spine and shoulders to the floor and proceed to bring your chin to your throat. Exhaling, tip the pelvis and slowly lower the small of the back, ribs, shoulder blades, and the back of your head to the mat.

Your entire back will, of course, *not* be on the mat. However, take 3 deep breaths on the exhalation, trying to tip the pelvis.

Relax in this flat Flounder pose, and let your muscles stretch out gradually. (The flounder is a very flat fish!) When you are comfortable, proceed.

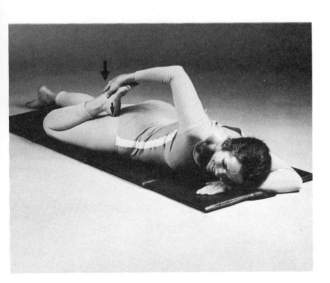

Frog

More Postures and Poses

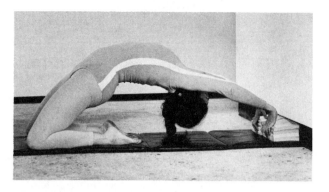

Flounder

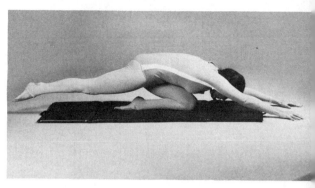

Nutcracker

Step 3

Place the hands, palms down, under your shoulders, fingertips facing the feet.

Inhale and press the heels of your hands into the mat. Exhale, push down, stretch your arms, tilt the pelvis, and raise your whole body, stretching the thighs and tightening the buttocks. Arch the entire spine and bend your elbows as you lower the top of your head to the floor. Lower your spine to the mat.

I personally find this arched Flounder difficult! My stiffness is in my shoulders. I have found it help-ful to place the heels of my hands on a high, thick book, which is secured against a wall or even the rung of a chair to achieve the necessary leverage for lifting the hips and thighs (see photo). (I also con-tinue persevering with shoulder-work exercises from chapter 5.)

To come out of this intense spine-and-groin stretch, it is imperative that you *do not* twist your back as you come up. Clasp the ankles firmly, squeeze the shoulders together, lift the head, press your weight evenly on both elbows and come up onto the elbows, sliding your hands down toward the toes. Then go beyond the toes. Place weight evenly on both hands and sit up. Relax in the Star pose, page 43.

NUTCRACKER

This strengthens and increases flexibility in thighs and ankles. Shoulder and chest muscles are fully exercised.

Kneel. Lean forward and place both hands on your mat. Your spine must be in a straight line. Your body forms a table.

Inhale then, exhaling, lift right leg up toward ceiling, keeping your hips level with floor. Lift the chin and sternum.

Inhale; then exhale. Try to hold the right leg as

high as possible as you lower your body onto the left thigh. Rest for a moment, stretching your right leg as far back as possible.

Now slide your body up to sit on your left heel. Place the left hand directly in front of your left knee on the mat for balance.

Inhale and lift sternum. Exhale, rotating the shoulders until the right shoulder is in line with your right thigh.

As you inhale, bend the right knee and reach down and grasp your right foot. Exhale, pull the right shoulder in and back, and tighten the right-buttock muscle, dropping your hip and bringing the right heel to touch your buttock. (Note photo.)

Work the shoulders in a straight line with your knee. Place the left hand on your left knee when you feel securely balanced.

As you hold this pose for 30 seconds, inhale while lifting up, and exhale as you work the foot close to the buttock. Then slowly come down and repeat on opposite side.

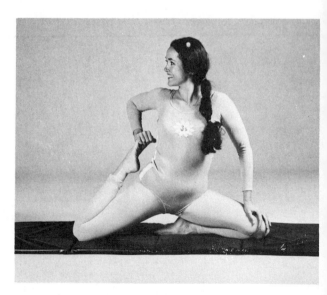

Nutcracker (heel touching buttocks)

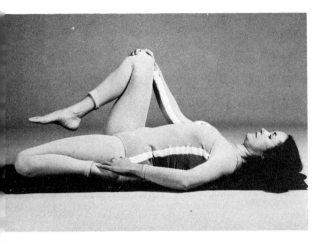

 Vise

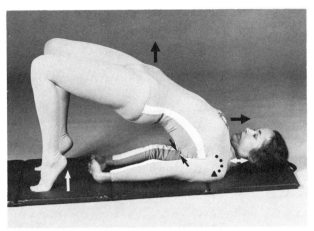

Bridge with Shoulder Rotation

VISE

A terrific stretch to your thighs, increasing flexibility to hips and feet. A good warmup for runners.

Step 1

Sit on your mat, legs straight out in front of you. Bend your right leg at the knee and bring the right foot beside (not under) your buttocks.

Lower your body weight down onto the elbows. Stop! Make sure that your right knee is on the floor. Rest in this position for 15 seconds. Inhale; then, exhaling, relax your knee and thigh muscles. Now bend your left leg and repeat the movements. Only when your left knee is to the mat should you continue to lower your back to the floor.

I would suggest you continue only when you feel comfortable and confident with Step 1.

Step 2

Inhale. Then as you exhale, try to tip the pelvis slowly. Bend the left knee and interlace your fingers around the lower left leg. Inhale, pulling shoulders down from the ears. Exhale and draw the left knee gently toward your chest. Take 3 deep breaths to relax and ease the knee closer.

To come out of this pose, straighten your left leg to the floor. Then turn onto your left elbow and then sit up.

Repeat the vise on the opposite leg.

BRIDGE WITH SHOULDER ROTATION

Lie on your back. Knees are bent, heels close to buttocks. As you raise the buttocks a few inches off the floor and slip your hands beneath the body, clasp your hands together, thumbs crossed. Straighten the elbows. Keep them on the mat. Inhale as you rotate the shoulders.

Come off the heels onto the balls of the feet and lift your hips up toward the ceiling. Exhaling, tip the pelvis.

Now work the shoulders more deeply in the posture as you use the stretching motion. Inhaling through the *nose*, open the chest deeply as you rotate the shoulders. Exhaling, tip the pelvis up higher on the balls of the feet. Repeat your rhythmical breath and stretch once more.

Now unclasp the hands. Note how the above movement has opened up the chest. Slowly return your spine to the floor; press down each individual vertebra, starting with the upper back, thus making the hips the very last to return to the floor. Then heels come back to the mat.

As you come down think to yourself *hips up, vertebra down*. It should take about 15 seconds to go up; hold 6 seconds; then return to the floor in 15 seconds. Breathe comfortably as you go through the up-and-down movement, and repeat Bridge with Shoulder Rotation 2 or 3 times.

Straighten your right and left legs. Relax and observe the sensation that follows.

Helpful Hints

Keep reminding yourself to check your knees. They should be 12 inches or hip-distance apart. It is much easier and safer on the cartilage!

Keep your knees, feet, and toes in a straight line.

FERRIS WHEEL

The Ferris Wheel strengthens your hands, increases flexibility of the spine, and tests your concentration.

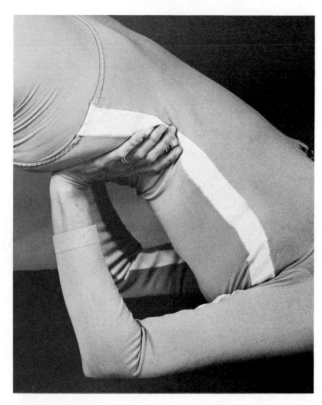

Ferris Wheel

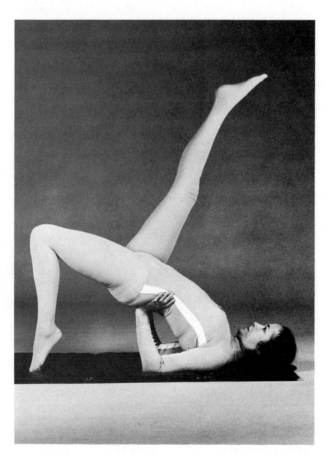

Ferris Wheel (Plow Pose)

Lie down on your back, knees bent, feet 12 inches apart (hip distance). Place your arms alongside the body, heels close to buttocks, and toes straight ahead.

Exhaling, tilt the pelvis; then slowly lift each vertebra off the mat.

Now reach both hands beneath you and rotate your shoulders. Clasp your hands together, intertwining fingers as if in prayer, thumbs crossing; straighten elbows. Keep the elbows straight, release the hands and push elbows into mat. Now place your wrists below your waist, cupping your lower back with your hand (note photo).

Inhale, lift the sternum and raise the right heel toward the ceiling as you lift the toes of the left foot.

Exhaling, complete the cycle as you now swing the right toes over the head to the mat. The left leg follows close behind as you bring the left foot over your head. (You are now in the Plow Pose.)

Pause briefly.

Inhale as you raise the left knee toward the ceiling, tightening both buttocks and extending the left hip forward. Now slowly lower the left foot to the floor. Let the right leg follow the left. You have completed 1 complete round of Ferris Wheel. Repeat 3 to 5 rounds each leg.

When through, place both feet on the floor and slowly come down to the mat one vertebra at a time. Tilt the pelvis and then relax. Take two Complete Breaths and then observe the body. Relax.

Helpful Hints

To lift the right leg all the way up and back, push off gently with the left toes. This is a light, rhythmical swing.

To maintain your lift, apply leverage into your ribs with hands and wrists. Elbows are directly under your hands.

DRAWBRIDGE

The Drawbridge is an exercise to help the flexibility of the entire spinal column, and also to firm, tone, and strengthen the front and back of the thighs.

Lie down, bend both knees, start with heels close to buttocks, arms alongside the body. Turn the palms upward. Pull the shoulders down from the ears.

Now slide the feet and ankles together. Inhale; then exhaling, tilt the pelvis and raise the right leg up toward the ceiling to the count of 5. Extend the heel of the right foot, kneecap pulled up.

Keep holding the right leg up. Inhale; then exhaling, press down the left foot, tilt the pelvis, raising the spine slowly off the mat 1 vertebra at a time. To maintain the height at the top of the pose, inhale and extend the sternum. Exhale, tightening the seat and tilting the pelvis. Hold to the count of 5.

Then still keeping the right leg raised, heel toward ceiling, lower your spine to the mat one vertebra at a time. Repeat 3 times on each leg.

The count is important in the Drawbridge. Raise the leg up *slowly* to the count of 5 and 1 second 1, 2 seconds 2, etc. Raise and lower the spine slowly to the count of 5, working up to 10.

Helpful Hints

Be sure the toes are pointing straight ahead and *not* out at an angle. The heels stay directly beneath the knees. The tibia, or shinbone, stays perpendicular to the floor.

When done correctly, the tightening of the buttocks and the extension of the sternum will alleviate lower-back tensions.

Remember to reward yourself with a good Relaxation Pose after the Drawbridge.

Execute this posture slowly.

Push down on the foot that is to the floor, but do not let the knee drift outward. This will help you to lift higher.

LOTUS POSES (PADMASANA)

Lotus poses pinpoint any ankle, knee, or hip stiffness. They align the spine; keep the mind attentive and alert; and encourage the natural curve of the spine. They are especially helpful for meditation and breathing.

Warmups

First warm up with all off-the-wall exercises, the Rock-a-Baby, and One Leg Forward Bend. "Retreat knees" (numb, or painful, stiff knees) are a common occurrence for beginners asked to sit for long periods of time. To help this problem, *do not* sit on the flat floor. I always elevate my hips by folding my mat (or blanket or high, firm pillow). My sitting bones (ischium) are at least 2 to 4 inches higher than my ankles. The elevation cants the spine forward. Also propping pillows beneath your knees will help support sore knee cartilage.

Technique 1

Sit tall on your folded blanket, legs straight out in front of you. Bend your right leg and place the right foot under your left knee. Bend your left leg, placing

your left foot under the right knee. Head and spine can be kept in a straight line in this comfortable easy pose.

Technique 2

Sit tall on your folded blanket. Bend your right leg and place the right heel up high against your left thigh. Bend the left leg and place the left foot *high* under the right leg.

Technique 3

This pose takes some getting used to, but it is far and away my most comfortable meditation pose.

Sit tall, reach down and bring your left foot up into the crotch. Bend your right leg and place your right foot in front of the left foot. The toes are along your shinbone.

Technique 4

Sit with your legs outstretched, bending your left leg at the knee. Place your left heel close to the crotch.

Then reach down, bend your right knee, holding your right foot with your hands and *turn* the sole of the foot to face you. Then place the right foot high on your left thigh. The right knee is close to the floor. The higher the heel toward your hip bone, the less pressure on the ankle.

Technique 5

Sit with your legs outstretched. Bend your left leg. Reach down and hold the left foot with your hands. Turn your foot so the sole is facing you. Place the left foot high on the right thigh as you lower the left knee to the mat.

Bend the right leg. Reach down and hold your

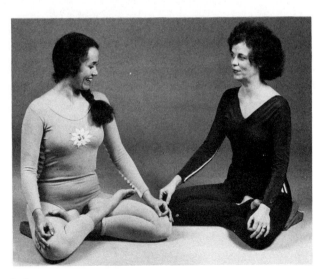

Lotus

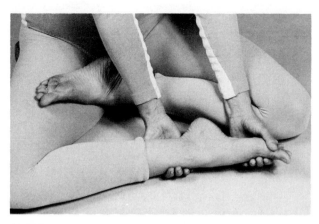
Half Lotus

right foot with your hands. Turn your sole. Then keep holding onto your instep with your left hand, but slip your right hand down to hold your ankle.

Draw your right foot in toward your folded left leg and lift the foot up just a few inches. Hold and observe. Does the lift cause you any discomfort? Go no farther than lifting up and placing the foot only 2 inches high on opposite leg. Never, never *yank* your foot up to your thigh. Gradually, inch by inch, bring the right foot higher up onto the folded left leg. Repeat the above process on the opposite leg.

Helpful Hints

Never force any position. Do spend time warming up well. Knee problems? Read more about knees in chapter 22, "Special Problems," page 171. It is natural to favor one side in Lotus, so remind yourself to reverse the process. Start with your stiff side first. Head, neck, and back are in alignment when in sitting poses. Bring your heel as close as possible to the crotch, or perineum. It is the exact center of your body. If at first your knees stick up like twin mountains, don't get discouraged. Practice will bring about results!

ABDOMINAL LIFT (UPPIYANA BANDHA)

This strengthens and keeps the abdominal muscles flexible. Also trims the waistline; relieves constipation and promotes regularity; tones and massages most abdominal organs and glands; improves circulation; and aids in digestion.

Please study all steps before working on this exercise.

Stand with your feet apart. Bend forward with knees bent. Place your hands on your thighs above the knees or wherever is most comfortable for you to get the most leverage.

Place the weight on your hands.

Exhale fully through your mouth. Close your mouth. Bring your chin to your throat and the tongue to roof of mouth. This vacuum is more easily experienced if you do a mock inhalation. You *do not* actually breathe at this point. The tongue acts as a lock to prevent air from coming in.

Relax the abdominal muscles. Draw the muscles in and upward as if your navel will touch your spine.

Hold inward for a second or two; then rhythmically snap the abdominal muscles in and out with a pull-in, release, pull-in, release, motion. Three to ? contractions are performed on one breath.

Do this 5 to 6 times. Inhale and stand up.

It is not unusual to have a coughing sensation after you complete this exercise.

Helpful Hints

Work up slowly from 5 to 25 lifts.

Exhale fully. It is the key to this exercise.

Remember tongue-lock. A relaxed abdomen permits the abdomen to hollow.

Practice in front of a mirror.

BEGINNER'S WHEEL (CHAKRASANA)

Strengthens and stretches hands and wrists. Opens the chest and tones the legs and seat. Excellent warmup for the more advanced Wheel pose.

Step 1

Sit on your mat, feet pointing straight ahead and hip distance apart (12 inches). Hands are behind you, fingertips facing wall behind your back.

Inhale, lifting your hips off the mat and dropping your head back. Squeeze shoulder blades together as you lift upward. This is the top of your pose.

Exhale. Lower the seat to floor. Head straight. Repeat 3 times.

Step 2

When you feel strong and confident in Step 1 go to the top of the pose. Inhale, lifting the left arm up toward the ceiling. Hold steadily. Exhale and lower to floor. Repeat on opposite side.

Repeat 3 times for each arm.

Step 3

Go to top of your pose. Inhale. Lift your right leg up, extending your heel; head stays back. Hold for 3 seconds. Exhale and bring the leg down and repeat on opposite leg.

Do 3 times for each leg.

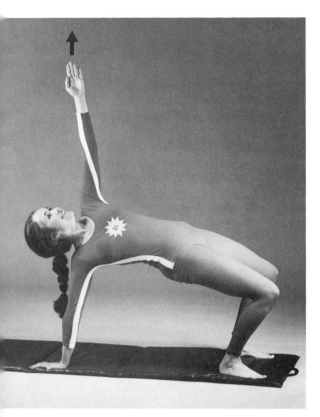

Beginner's Wheel (Step 2)

WHEEL

I enjoy working with this pose directly on the floor. Bare feet are an absolute *must*. Socks slip! Please work often with the Flounder, the Bridge pose, the Fish Over a Barrel, and the Beginner's Wheel for 3 months; then try the Wheel.

The Wheel is a terrific strengthener for the arms and legs. It also increases spinal flexibility, tones the abdomen and thighs, and energizes your nervous system. It's a marvelous release of tensions!

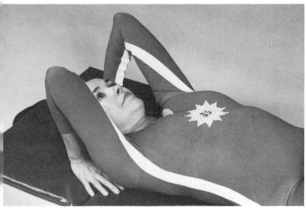

Wheel (Step 1)

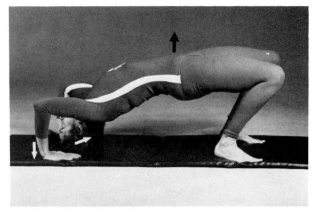

Wheel (hips lifted, spine arched)

Step 1

Lie down, bend your knees, clasp the ankles, and bring the heels close to your buttocks. Place your hands palms down, fingertips under the shoulders. Please note my hand position.

Inhale, extend the sternum, tighten the buttocks, and lift your hips as you come onto your shoulders. Exhale, coming to the crown (top) of your head. The spine is arched. (Note photo.)

Before going any further, go through this mental checklist:

1. Feet parallel, 12 inches apart?
2. Knees directly above the feet?
3. Are the heels of the hands pressed against the floor?
4. Are the fingertips pointing toward the feet?
5. Am I able to push down on the heels of my hands to lift my head off the floor with moderate ease?

If the answer to number 5 is, "No, I'm afraid," or "it's *impossible* for me to straighten my elbow," then don't proceed beyond Step 1 for a few weeks. Don't try to force the arms straight! Let your entire body become adjusted slowly and continue to work on your upper-back flexibility by doing the Fish Over a Barrel.

Step 2

Inhale. Extend the sternum and tighten the buttocks. Lead with the sternum as you exhale, pushing against the heels of the hands, straightening the arms while the head raises from the floor smoothly. Your neck is relaxed.

Step 3

Come off the heels of your feet onto the ball of the foot. Inhale, tightening the buttocks as you tilt

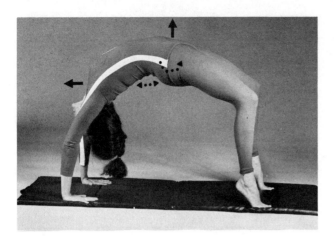

Wheel (Step 3)

the pelvis and flatten the abdomen. Hips are lifting toward the ceiling.

Exhale and, using the balls of your feet for leverage, gently push your sternum forward toward the wall you are facing. Repeat this inhalation–hips up–exhalation 3 times. This up and forward motion will keep the lower-lumbar vertebrae as free as possible from compression.

To come down, return the tip of your head to the floor (as in Step 1); then touch the chin to your chest and bring the shoulders and spine to the floor. Relax in a knee-to-chest position.

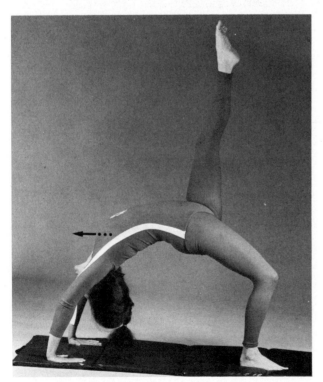

Wheel (leg lifts)

Variation 1

Go through the preceding Steps 1 and 2. Hold at top of Step 2. To maintain your balance, adjust the hands by sliding your right hand slightly into the center. Inhale; then exhaling move your right foot slightly toward the center. Then inhale and raise your left leg up toward the ceiling or extend the heel or point your toe. Hold; then lower it to the floor. Repeat on the opposite side.

Variation 2

If you feel confident and challenged, go to the top of the Wheel. Slide your right hand slightly into the center for balance. Inhale, then exhaling slowly lift the left arm up toward the ceiling and place it on your left thigh. Then lower the left hand to the floor and repeat with right arm. Remain in pose for the 3 deep breaths, always pushing your sternum forward to wall behind you. Then come out of pose and rest. Breathe deeply, and tell yourself what a great job you've just done, because it's true! Then turn on your left side, sit up, and go into the Star pose, page 43.

SUN SALUTATION (SURYA NAMASKAR)

This beautiful, flowing, twelve-part exercise has long been a favorite of mine. It is a wonderful warm-up and a great way to get creaking bones moving early in the morning; moreover, insomniacs will find that after 6 to 8 rounds, tensions are worked out and sleep is possible.

This exercise improves overall body circulation, increases stamina and energy, and makes the spine supple and healthy. It also reduces the waist and abdomen.

For the Sun Salutation, consider the sun as the symbol of glowing health and vital energy. As you go through each motion, visualize yourself basking in its life-giving vibration no matter what the weather is outside your window.

Repeat this exercise 4 to 12 times.

1. Stand with your feet together. Feet are lined up with the lines on the floor. Tighten your knee-caps, tilt the pelvis, palms together over your heart center (chest). Shoulders down from ears.
2. Inhale, raising the arms above the head. Contract the buttocks muscles *firmly*; lift the sternum toward the ceiling; and keep your head between the upper arms. Lift your torso upward as you lean back. Pause. Hold for only 3 seconds.

Lilias, Yoga, and Your Life

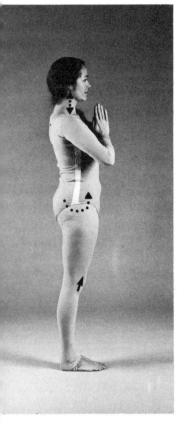 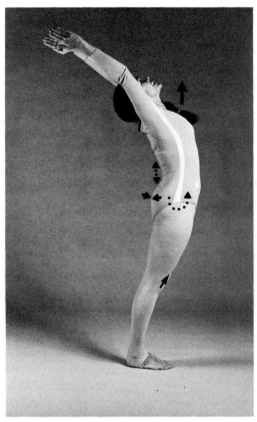 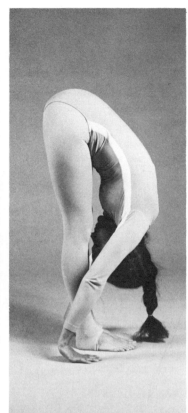

Posture 1 Sun   Sun Salutation (Technique I) (Step 2)

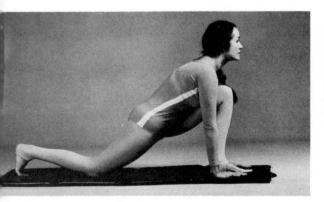 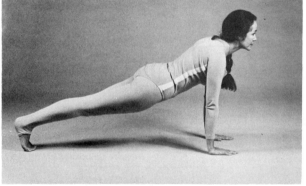

Sun Salutation (Technique I) (Step 3)   Sun Saluation (Technique I) (Step 4)

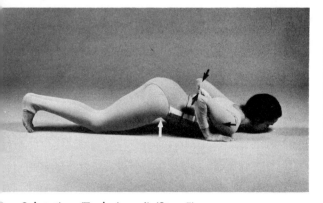 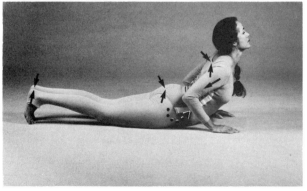

Sun Salutation (Technique I) (Step 5)   Sun Salutation (Technique I) (Step 6)

3. Exhale and reaching out, extend your arms forward and down to floor. Knees straight. If you are limber, bring your fingertips on either side of the toes to form one line of nails. Do not move your hands from this position until you raise them for Step 11. Lower the ribs, chest to your thighs.

4. Bend both knees and place your hands flat on the floor on either side of the feet. Slide your right foot as far back as you can go. Right knee is on the mat. This is similar to a Lunge (page 103).

5. Now slide your left foot back alongside the right foot. In body-straight position. Pull the stomach in. Hold your breath, or breathe shallowly.

6. Exhale and bend both knees to the mat; arch your spine, hips up in the air, elbows close to your body. Lower the chest and chin to the mat. Pause 3 to 5 seconds.

7. Using the toes for leverage, push (or shoot) your chest 6 inches beyond, between the thumbs. Then, inhaling, raise forehead, nose, chin, chest, and ribs, arching your back in a modified Cobra. Keep your hips and navel on the mat! The upper neck is relaxed. Pause 3 to 5 seconds.

8. Curl your toes under; raise the hips up to the ceiling until the arms and legs are straight. Exhale, pushing against the heels of your hands and leaning the weight into the heels of your feet. Look at your feet. Do not force the head to the floor. This position is called the Dog.

9. Shift your weight to the left foot and left hand as you bring your right foot up forward to line up with fingers once again. Inhale and look up, chin raised, left knee on the mat.

10. Exhale and *push off* with the toes of your left foot. (Do not drag your foot up.) Bring the left foot up to the right. Place palms of hands on either side of your feet, or simply bring the hands forward, arms relaxed. Do not bounce. Let the weight of your upper body bring you forward.

11. Inhale and reach out toward the wall in front of you. Then continue raising the arms up to the ceiling. Raise your kneecaps. (Watch for overextended knees.) Exhale and tighten the buttocks. Keep your head between your upper arms. Now, once again, inhale and lift the sternum up toward the ceiling. Keep lifting and tightening buttocks as you go back! Pause only 3 seconds.

12. Exhale and return to a standing pose. Repeat on opposite leg.

Details and Comments

Fainting in a Yoga class is not a common occurrence, but it sometimes *does* happen. It usually i caused by a student's forgetting to take a deep breath before going into arches or backward bends. Therefore, take special care to inhale totally before you go from Position 1 into 2 and 10 into 11. Hold the arch only 3 seconds; then go into Position 3 or Position 12.

In Position 2, it is easy to compress the lumbar vertebra as you go into the bend; therefore, tighten the buttocks muscles to protect your lower back. No pain is to be felt in the number 2 pose. Keep the torso lifted throughout this bend. Think of number 2 *not* as an arc, but rather a bend.

In Position 3, relax your face as you hold this pose. Let the cheeks flow over your eyes and the weight of the head pull you forward. Do not bounce. Bend your knees slightly if the back of the legs bother you, or bend them-straighten them 6 times to loosen them up.

In Position 4, the right knee is not in front of the toes of your right foot. The right knee and lower leg form a 90-degree angle with the floor. The palms of your hands are flat to the floor. Do not balance on your thumbs!

In Position 5, do not sag in this body-straight pose. Stomach in. Your head is up. It is an extension of the spine. If you have arthritic wrists, balance on the knuckles of your clenched fist or on lower arms.

In Position 6, the arms and chest are at first weak; and going from 5 to 6 can be literally a big flop for beginners. Therefore, keep the elbows *close* to your body for strength. Also, it is perfectly okay to learn this position from your mat. In other words, from 5 body straight pose place the body flat onto the mat. Then go into knee, and chin position. As you become stronger, 5 will flow into 6 with ease. In Position 6, your hips should form a tunnel high enough for a rabbit to go through, but *not* an elephant!

In Position 7, tilt your pelvis for lower-back protection.

In Position 8, while in the Dog, work within the pose. Use your breath to help you rhythmically elongate and lengthen.

As you go from *Position 9* into *Position 10*, do not allow your right foot to drag as your bring it up to *Position 10*. Too sloppy! Push off with your toes. This gives you added strength and fineness.

Variations on the Sun Salutation

I have always enjoyed creating variations on a theme of Sun Exercise. You too can make up your own movements. These variations are for the stu-

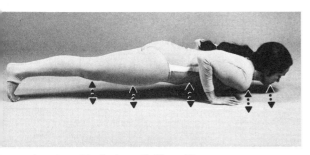

Sun Salutation (Technique I) (Step 7)

lent who knows Sun inside and out, and has a degree of flexibility!

Position 1 Raise your arms up to the ceiling and inhale. Stretch fingers upward. Lift out of the rib cage. Exhale and sway to your right. Repeat on your left.

Position 2 Chest Expander. Clasp your hands behind you. Straighten the elbows; tighten the buttocks. Inhale and lift your chin, arms, and sternum up toward the ceiling.

Position 3 Exhale, still in Chest Expander, bend forward, leading with the chin, hands clasped above your head. Bring your face toward the knees. Release your hands.

Position 4 With the right leg back, lift your right knee 2 inches off mat. Hold 10 seconds. Palms flat.

Position 5 Lower your straight body to 4 inches off the mat. Hold 5 to 10 seconds, breathing shallowly.

Position 6 Inhale and raise your right leg. Exhale and lower. Repeat on left leg.

Position 7 In Cobra, look over the right shoulder. Then slowly look over your left shoulder.

Position 8 The Dog. Inhale and lift right leg up to the ceiling. Exhale, leg down to floor. Repeat on left leg.

Position 9 Lift your chest off your right thigh. Place arms in T position. Twist the shoulders to the right; then twist back to center. Place palms together. Inhale, arch the back, tighten your right buttock. Return to original position.

Position 10 Standing Forward Bend. Bend the knees. Reach around behind your knees and grab the elbows. Press your chest to your thighs. Now bend knees, bringing knees close to your cheekbones. Then gently straighten them. Repeat 6 times. Thighs stay tight to your chest. Still keeping the thighs glued to your chest, inhale; then lower the arms down your calves, elongating and breathing into this deep stretch.

Position 11 With feet 3 feet apart, bend your knees. Now push the knees, thighs, and pelvis forward beyond the feet. Tighten your buttocks *firmly*. Place your hands on the upper-thigh muscles, slightly below the buttocks, for leverage. Squeeze your shoulders and elbows together. Inhale. Hips forward, look to your back wall, lift the sternum, drop the head back. *Keep breathing* and lifting as you hold 10 seconds. No lower back pain!

Position 12 Stand with your feet together, arms relaxed. Relax the shoulders; close the eyes. Inhale, breathing in energy and lightness. Exhale all fatigue, tension and darkness! Repeat inhaling all that is positive; exhaling all negatives. Repeat and really feel that you are ready to accept health and well-being as you inhale. As you exhale, feel and imagine yourself surrendering all uneasiness of body, mind, and spirit.

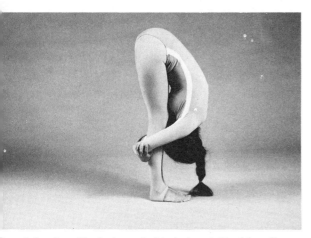

Sun Saluation (Technique I) (Variations) (Position 5)

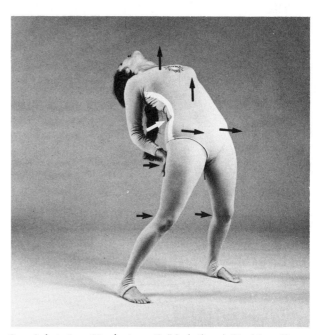

Sun Saluation (Technique I) (Variations) (Position 2)

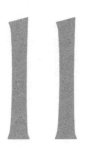

Basic Getting-Started Routines and Practice Schedules

I think it's a help for you to have a schedule that tells you what follows what, and how to add on safely, week by week.

After you have read the chapters on breathing, relaxation, and building blocks, start this half-hour routine each day for 2 to 4 weeks. Do these routines in the following order:

First and Second Weeks

Neck Tilt
Neck Rolls
Elbow Pull
Push Away
Chicken Wings
Hulk
All shoulder work exercises
Side Rock-and-Roll
Any two tension relievers from chapter 3
Pelvic Tilt
Single Leg Raise
Single Leg Raise with Tie
Rest—three Complete Breaths
Forehead-to-Knee pose, page 127, chapter 16
One Leg Forward Bend with Twist
Easy Twist, page 127, chapter 16
Mecca Pose

Standing Toe Lift
Rag Doll
Standing Side-to-Side Pose
Six rounds of Complete Breath
Five-minute Relaxation
Start reading directions for Leg Raises and chapter 13, "Back Talk"

Third Week

Add:
Windmill
Space Walk
Pendulum Leg Swing
Side Leg Lifts 1 and 2
Dog
Cat Arch
Arm Leg Lifts 1 and 2
Slant Board, page 94, chapter 13
Spinal Warmups 1 and 2
Read chapter 12, "Creative Stress—Creative Tension"
Reread pages on relaxation and breathing

Fourth Week

Add:
Neck Ups
Sitback
Standing Lunge (with a chair)
Chest Expander
Eagle
Triangle
Read chapter 15, "Sitting Fit"

This routine should get your Hatha Yoga practice started. Please take your time. Have fun. Be patient with yourself. I've used *weeks* only for clarity and organization's sake. If it takes you 2 months, that's fine!

FIVE-MINUTE YOGA ROUTINE
Sun Salutation—Start with 4, work up to 8; then, in a matter of months, 6 to 12
Lie down, 10 Complete Breaths
Relaxation—3 minutes.

TWENTY-MINUTE YOGA ROUTINE
Sun Salutation—4 to 6 times
Rest—take 6 Complete Breaths
Rock-a-Baby

Dolphin—hold 30 seconds to 1 minute
Forehead to Knee
Half-Candle—hold 30 seconds; work up to 3 minutes; after 2 months, Full Shoulderstand
Windmill
Fish
Sitback
Cobra
Neck Up
Forward Bend—hold 1 minute
Easy Twist
Dragon Breath
Relaxation

THIRTY-MINUTE ROUTINE

Neck Roll
Knees Side by Side
Legs in V Position 1 and 2
Intermediate Leg Stretch
Cat Arch
Dog Wag
Hydrant
Sun Salutation 2 to 4
Chest Expander
Stomach Lift
Crocodile
Dog Stretch
Locust Warmups 1 and 2
Sky Diver
Mecca
Flying Bird (Garud Asana)
Practice 1 posture you do not enjoy doing; then practice your favorite pose
Cleansing Breath
Relaxation

Your Morning Routine

Stepping stone warmups
Stretch and Yawn
Standing Side-to-Side Sway
Rag Doll
Forehead to Knee
Foot Flaps
Neck-and-Shoulder Rolls
Neck Tilt and Neck Up
Space Walk
Windmill
Knees Side to Side
Rest and take 3 Complete Breaths
Side Rock and Roll
Bridge with Shoulder Rotation
Wheel
Dancer's Pose

2 Sitbacks
Asanas with their corresponding warmups
2-4-6 Sun Salutations
Spinal Walking
Cobra
Sky Diver
Bow
One Leg Forward Bend
Forward Bend
Mecca Pose
Pendulum Leg Swing
Crocodile
Abdominal Lift
Leg Lunge
Triangle Pose
Flying Bird (Garud Asana)
Wall Lean
Cleansing Breath
5 minutes of Relaxation

Your Evening Routine
(approximately forty-five minutes)

Tense and Hold
Stretch and Yawn
Rack
Neck Tilt
Lemon Squeeze
Rock-and-Roll
Cat Arch
Torso Twist
Dog Wag
Hydrant
Mecca Pose
Rag Doll
Chest Expander, work up to arm movement
Standing Side to Side
Half-Moon Standing
Rest and take 3 to 6 Complete Breaths
2-6-8 Moon Salutations or 2-6-8 Sun Salutations
Rest and take 6 Complete Breaths
Dolphin, hold 30 seconds
Half Candle or Full Shoulderstand for 1 minute or longer
Fist—15 seconds
Forward Bend for 1 to 3 minutes
Inclined Plane (with arm raise)
Triangle Pose
Practice 1 posture you do not enjoy; then practice your favorite pose
Dragon Breath
4 to 10 rounds of Complete Breath
5 to 10 minutes of Relaxation

Stretch and Strengthen Routine—Intermediate Level

Dancer's Pose
Intermediate Crossed Ankle Rock and Roll
Sitback (with arm variations)
Staff
12 Sun Salutations—6 slowly, paying attention to breath, 6 quicker flowing movements
Plow—1 to 3 minutes
Shoulderstand—work up to 3 minutes; then leg variations
Headstand—up to 3 minutes
Fish—30 seconds
Rest—3 to 6 Complete Breaths
Forward Bend—3 to 5 minutes
Crocodile
Dragon Breath
Shield
Flying Bird (Garudasana)
Eagle
Wheel—start work on leg lifts
Rest 15 to 30 seconds in Star
10 rounds of Complete Breath with positive suggestions
Relaxation—5 minutes

You have now done a day's schedule.

Here are a few postures with their appropriate strengthening exercises. Not all postures have been included. You the student, make up your own creative list; these are just examples.

In preparing for Standing Poses, the following strengtheners are helpful:

Off-the-wall exercises; all shoulder work; Foot Flaps; Neck Ups; Neck Tilt; Rock-a-Baby; Dancer's V Pose; all Leg Raises; Sitback with Arms; Star; Half-Moon Standing; Standing Side to Side; One Leg Forward Bend; One Leg Forward Bend with Twist; Lunge Warmup.

For the Cobra, the following warmups and strengtheners are appropriate:

All shoulder work; Spinal Warmups 1 to 2; Skydiver; Windmill; Push Ups 1 to 3; Neck Tilt; Neck Ups; and Space Walk. Be sure also to read the chapter on Back Talk.

For the Bow the following warmups and strengtheners are appropriate:

Foot Flaps; Locust Warmups; Maltese Cross; Spinal Warmups; Cobra; Lemon Squeeze; Bridge with Shoulder Rotation; Pelvic Tilt; and all shoulder work.

For the Full Shoulderstand, the following warmups and strengtheners are appropriate:

Neck Tilt; Neck Ups; Crossed Ankle Rock and Roll; Side Rock and Roll; Forehead to Knee; Sitbacks with arms; Maltese Cross; Bridge with Shoulder Rotation; Double-Heel Descent; Push Ups; Space Walk; Intermediate Leg Stretch; and the emotional stability routine.

For the Beginner's Fish, the following warmups and strengtheners are appropriate:

Spinal Warmups 1–3; Neck Ups; Neck Tilt; Fish Over a Barrel; Leg Raises; Bridge with Shoulder Rotation; Lemon Squeeze; and all shoulder work.

The following warmups and strengtheners are appropriate for the headstand:

Dolphin with Head Raises; Push Ups 1–3; Leg Raises; Sitback; Neck Ups; Tilt the Pelvis; Over-the-Head Arm Clasp; Standing Balance Poses for self-confidence; and Cobra and Bow (flexibility of spine).

For the Forward Bend, the following are appropriate:

Off the Wall; Hip Rotation Against Wall; Crossed Ankle Rock and Roll; Forward Bend Using Book and Belt; Pendulum; Rock-a-Baby; Single Leg Raises with Belt; Windmill; Side Rock and Roll; Spinal Warmups; Twist; and Leg Lifts.

For the Plough, the following are appropriate:

Hip Rotation with Wall or Chair; Neck Ups; Two-Arm Lemon Squeeze; Crossed Ankle Rock and Roll; all Forward Bends; Forehead-to-Knee pose; and Rock-a-Baby.

For the Spider, the following are appropriate:

Intermediate Leg Stretch; Wall U; Intermediate Rock and Roll; and One Leg Forward Bend.

The following warmups are appropriate for the Camel:

Neck Ups and Fish.

For the Flounder, the following are appropriate:

Neck Ups; Bridge; Beginner's Wheel; Forehead to Knee; Fish Over a Barrel; and Spinal Warmup.

For the Wheel Pose, the following warmups and strengtheners are appropriate:

Side Rock and Roll; Crossed Ankle Rock and Roll; Leg Lifts; Sitbacks; Pelvic Tilt; Neck Ups; all shoulder work; Spinal Warmups; Cobra; Flounder; Bridge with Shoulder Rotation; Drawbridge; Kneeling Bridge; Fish Over a Barrel; Beginner's Wheel with Leg Lifts; Forward Bends; Vise; Nutcracker, and Frog.

Now we come to the chapter which has been the most difficult for me to write. I am sure this is because the subject matter is so close to the nerve endings of my life now and for many years to come. This chapter is by no means finished—it is a beginning.

Let me start by sharing this little story with you. When relaxation is finished at the end of class, there is a very special feeling in the room. It is hard to describe. It is conveyed through gentle smiles, quiet eyes, and serene faces.

But one day, many years ago, it was different. I spotted a woman sitting on her mat looking forlorn and fearful. I walked over and asked her what she was feeling and would talking help. She looked up; disappointment ringed her eyes.

"Everyone else looks so happy. Why do I feel so sad? So scared? Perhaps it's because you asked me to let go of my heavy emotional baggage, and I wanted to keep holding on. Tension and stress in my life are the glue that holds me together. Without it, I almost feel lonely, or that I'll just fall apart."

I had few words of comfort to give her. I'd never seen a student experience this before. As I watched her leave, I felt disappointed at not being able to help her. She never returned to class. Her questions left a lasting impression upon me.

Only after years of teaching did I realize that my immaturity as a teacher, asking the students blithely to give up "their tension" without delving more positively beneath the surface, had kept me from helping her. It took me years to truly understand that tension will be with us all until the day we take our last breath, and that it is vital to our creativity. Even in meditation there is tension, but it is in better balance. Negative stress and negative tensions, which are the by-products of negative emotions, deplete the energy, produce toxins within the body, twist and cramp the mind.

OBSERVATION

Yoga teachers of the past and present feel that stressful emotions such as fear, bitterness, anger, envy, jealousy, resentment, self-pity, depression and hate are all very toxic energy that take on special forms and attach themselves to and crystalize within the internal organs and joints of the body. This toxicity is thought to increase the risk of heart attack, cancer, high blood pressure, ulcers, diabetes, arthritis, and even accidents. We have the ability to project these destructive, poisonous forces through a

12
Creative Stress— Creative Tension

glance, through our voices, our words, and other ways of expression.

Negative and stressful emotions should *not* be suppressed because hiding them is unhealthy and dangerous. One method I have found extremely helpful is training yourself to detach and observe and not identify with emotions. You can release yourself from their control without harming others.

If you were going to shave or put on make-up, and the mirror was misty, would you press your nose against the glass to see? Of course not. You'd pull

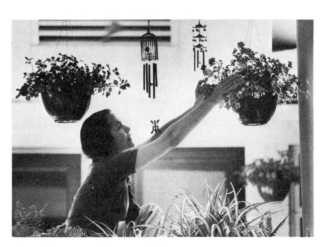

Creative Stress (Lilias with flowers)

back, "making space" between you and the reflected image. You would then wipe off the mirror, take a clear look, and become the OBSERVER, observing the reflection of your face.

Developing your witness-self takes time and practice. It is a tool I use daily. At first I just watched myself make my bed, wash a dish, or brush my teeth. As I began to observe the feeling and sensation within my own body during and after the exercise and relaxation, the witness-self became clearer. Then, after more time, I could observe or watch my moments of irritability or laziness or impatience. Once I saw these moods, I could *do* something positive about them.

DETACHMENT

The word *detachment* is probably one of the most misunderstood words in all of Yoga and esoteric teachings. Detachment does not mean lack of interest or losing your connection with reality. Nor does it mean cool aloofness. And detachment does not mean rejection! "Detachment produces the serenity of releasing to embrace, while rejection produces pain, anguish and let-me-out-of-here feelings."* Detachment is a mature attitude or state or mind.

Perhaps the most difficult obstacle to attaining this healthy detached attitude is learning not to judge, not to criticize what you observe within *yourself*. If we can first train ourselves to unemotionally observe objects in a room, parts of the body, and then our thinking process, we are a step closer to training ourselves to observe our emotional self and our feeling self without judgments.

As you achieve dispassionate, noncritical detachment, you are no longer under judgment's illusion. You have transmuted and transferred this toxic energy into something higher and positive. The misty mirror then becomes a clearer reflection. The darkness is transmuted into light; anger into acceptance; jealousy into self-esteem; hate into love.

I too struggle hard with detaching myself from old feelings, old relationships and memories. It has been a little like looking into my clothes closet, which bulges with outdated clothes from fifteen years ago. I can't seem to throw them out. Just as I am unable to give up or let go the unworn clothes, so my mind has difficulty releasing past memories, negative judgments, criticisms, worries about the

* W. Brugh Joy, M.D. *Joy's Way* (Los Angeles, CA: J. P. Tarcher, Inc. 1979).

future. Releasing them through an active positive meditation or the *Seven Steps to Effective Prayer* (page 5) is a little like the process of rolling up my sleeves and cleaning out my closet. When I do it, I feel lighter in all directions and on many levels.

We will never rid ourselves of our emotional self, nor do we wish to. It is like an ocean that surrounds us. What we wish to do is calm the ocean's waves by controlling, organizing, and transmuting the energy from negative stress to a positive tension. Just as we begin to control the physical body by using purer food, exercising and breathing, so can we calm the ocean of our emotional body with the following simple techniques.

THE ART OF DETACHMENT—PART I

I wish to extend special thanks to H. Saraydarian, author of *The Science of Becoming Oneself*, for some of the exercises found in this chapter.

Technique 1: Eyes Open Observation

Sit or lie down. Open your eyes and look carefully around you. Notice the colors, lines, angles, fixtures of the wall, ceiling, furniture, rug and lamps. If your mind wanders, refocus it on the objects you are seeing. Remind yourself you are the observer who is witnessing the room. Try this exercise for one minute each morning and evening.

Technique 2: Daily Observation

Observe or witness yourself as you do everyday actions, such as getting dressed, washing the dishes, driving the car, riding the subway or commuter train, talking on the phone, making the bed, walking down the street.

Technique 3: Sleep Observation

Observe as you go through the relaxation process. After you've spent one month on the above exercises, proceed with Technique 4.

Technique 4: Listen and Visualize

Sit and listen to a portion of some fine music, such as Beethoven's *Eighth Symphony* or Rachmaninoff's *Concerto No. 2 in C Minor*. Take a few calming breaths. Keep the music on as you imagine you are sitting in some favorite spot in the country. Visualize the flowers, the grass, the water, the rocks. Now dig deeply into yourself to visualize clearly the colors, the sounds and the shapes. Hold yourself in

Lilias, Yoga, and Your Life

this lovely place of peace and tranquility for five to ten minutes; then listen to the balance of the piece of music. Practice this each day for three weeks; then proceed to Technique 5.

Technique 5: Dance Fantasy

Again listen to a piece of fine music. Use your imagination and go to any lovely place you wish. Visualize dancers performing to the rhythm of this beautiful music. Be free of previous concepts of dance (folk or ballet); create a dance fantasy of graceful angel-like dancers moving, gliding magically around. Bring forth all the colors of the rainbow and the combinations of colors, light, and forms. Invent more creative and intricate dance and light patterns, all taking place within one large picture frame.

After you have visualized this for some minutes, return listening to the music until it ends. At first, your visualization will be weak but as with muscles it will be strengthened with practice. Do the above set of exercises for at least six weeks before you start Part II.

THE ART OF DETACHMENT—PART II

At first you might find these exercises repugnant and difficult. This is understandable. They are meant to clean out our emotional vehicle of negative stress and negative emotions. It takes courage and practice to look squarely at these emotions. Please do them slowly, and in the order recommended. They are especially devised to strengthen the observer within you and to develop your powers of healthy detachment.

Technique 1: Cockfight, or Birds Fighting

Once a day during the first week relax your body, take two deep slow breaths, play some lovely music, go to your special place of nature. Now imagine two birds fighting. Allow them to fight fiercely, pecking, clawing, screaming at each other. They pull feathers and have bloody wounds. Witness this scene; then sit quetly until the music stops. Observe if you've been able to witness this scene without emotion, as the indifferent observer.

Technique 2: Animals Fighting

Once a day during the second week, go back to the same music and scene, but this time visualize two animals fighting. Follow the same procedure as the indifferent observer.

Technique 3: Listening to Gossip

Once a day the third week imagine a person (man or woman) starting ugly, malicious gossip about someone you love; then watch the same person start malicious gossip about someone you dislike; and then about someone to whom you are indifferent. Observe yourself listening very calmly, very quietly, with a detached attitude.

Technique 4: Observing Negative Emotions

For the next 4 weeks imagine a drama, using one negative emotion from those on page 83. Using anger, for example, imagine the entire motions of an angry person and then watch yourself as if you were watching another person. (If the word *anger* is too difficult for you to observe, then start with another word that is less charged from your point of view.)

Starting in the fifth week give yourself the starring role as you continue creating dramas. But, for each of the listed emotions remember to observe him or her and with no feeling of identification, judgment or criticism. You are the observer observing yourself!

THE ART OF DETACHMENT—PART III

Negative thoughts and emotions punctuate our thinking and everything around us. They affect our body chemistry in ways that prepare us for muscular action or stressful situations. Therefore, it is of the utmost importance that, as you see your expressed negative emotions, you have a technique to deal with them. Here is one of many ways.

Sit in a chair, relax your body, take a deep slow Complete Breath, and close your eyes. Now begin to re-enact the scene or experience. Suppose you are with a group of people who have been stingingly critical of you. Even after many months, you still feel the hurt. You have reacted with negative words and negative inner dialogue. Re-create the entire event in your mind.

But this time, imagine a perfect being of your "ideal teacher" sitting in front of you. Visualize yourself giving this perfected being the full extent of your black feelings. As the teacher receives this into his or her hands, watch the substance burst into light. The energy has been transformed into good— something higher. Then *thank* all the persons who have voiced the criticism. Giving thanks for our so-called problems is *another* way to transmute the problem energy.

As we identify ourselves less with emotion and

more with the transformation or the light, we shall find that we will dominate *it*, rather than the negative tension and emotion dominating us.

All the exercises in this chapter are extremely valuable. Put them to work immediately. Very soon, you will feel a new energy and optimism flow throughout your being. You will radiate a new spirit of tolerance and understanding and best of all you will feel a new love of self and of others.

CREATIVE STRESS

In this chapter we have learned specific mental exercises on how to work creatively with our stress and tensions. The following exciting, yet demanding set of sequential Yoga postures, when learned, will take you only fifteen minutes to do. You'll feel lighter, calmer, happier, and you'll experience a definite quieting of all inner mental dialogue.

This intriguing Emotional Stability Routine (ESR) is a combination of 12 Yoga postures done in quick, yet smooth succession. The Yoga teachers of old knew instinctively that negative tensions and emotions, constant inner dialogue, were woven into the respiratory process. They understood that our respiratory machinery was designed so that we could deliberately alter, disrupt and correct shallow, irregular breathing so often associated with depression or gloomy feelings.

ESR is designed for people who lack willpower and a decisive quality to their character. It will have an immediate and significant effect on your autonomic nervous system. It is well worth your effort.

I suggest you learn it in steps, taking Steps 1–9 every day for a few weeks. Then add on 10–20, and then do 1–28. The form does not have to be perfect, but don't flop through each exercise! Please pay attention to the breathing sequence.

The following routine will help you break out of old, negative thought patterns and depression. It will tone and strengthen your abdominal muscles. New strength within the body will help you become physically resistant to emotional stress and strain. You should perspire, and your lungs should be working hard after Steps 1–26.

My gratitude and thanks to the teachers of The Light of Yoga Society, Cleveland, Ohio, who shared this series of exercises with me.

Techniques 1–4: Standing Pendulum
1. Start standing with hands on hips. Place feet 3 feet apart.

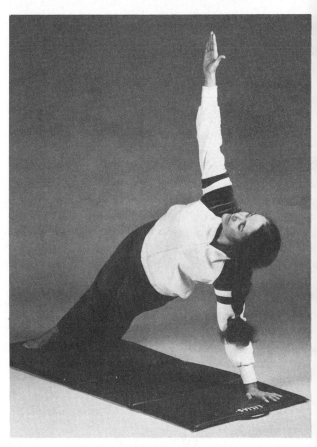

Plank (No. 8)

2. Inhale; then, exhaling, lower your head down toward the right knee; then go to the left knee. Inhale, and come back to your start position.
3. Repeat to left side.
4. Exhale in a half circle left; inhale and make a circle to your right. Repeat 6 times each side.

Techniques 5–6: Cobra to Dog
Place your hands and knees on the mat. Hands in line with shoulders; knees in line with hips.

Exhale and jacknife the hips toward ceiling into Dog Stretch; then inhale and go down to small Cobra. Your hips are 3 inches off the mat. Arms are straight. (Caution. Do not thrust weight into your lower back in this exercise even though you are moving quickly. Remember to tilt the pelvis.) Repeat 5 to 6 times.

Technique 7: Plank
Do once on each side. Hold for 5 to 10 seconds.

Place your hands directly beneath your body, parallel to mat; shoulders and legs are straight; and toes are tucked under to mat. Inhaling, lift your right arm out in front of you, breathing shallowly. Hold for 5 seconds.

Techniques 8–20

8. Turn and raise your right arm up toward ceiling. Your feet form a straight line, toes pointing right to the floor. Hold for 5 seconds, breathing shallowly. Return both hands to mat. Repeat on the opposite arm.

9. Relax curled up in Pose of a Child (page 92). Knees are bent, and your hands are alongside the body. Forehead to floor.

10. Again place your hands and knees on the mat. Inhale.

11. Then exhaling, round your spine and draw your right knee to forehead.

12. Inhaling, raise your right leg toward ceiling, chin up!

13–14. Exhaling keep your right leg up, lower your chin and chest to your mat, elbows out. (You should be able to balance on your right knee in this pose. It is not a pushup!) Inhaling do number 12 again and then exhaling repeat entire procedure 11–14 again, 6 times for each leg.

15. Rest in the Pose of a Child.

16. Come up to a sitting position. Knees are bent, feet are flat to the floor, and your hands are flat alongside your hips. Inhale.

17. Exhaling, round your spine, using your hands for leverage and balance. Roll back, bringing your feet over your head into the Plow. Keep the legs straight. Pause.

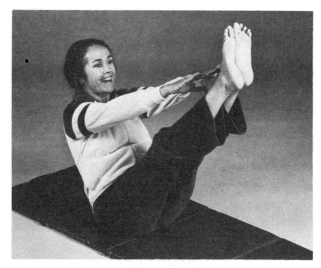

Big Situp (No. 21)

18. Then start the inhalation. Lower your legs back down to the floor. Finish inhaling and pause.

19. Then start exhaling as you push down on your hands. Bring your feet over your head to Plow. Finish exhaling when toes finally touch behind your head.
17–19 are smooth, quick-flowing movements. Do this Plow 6 times.

20. Rest. Take 6 complete breaths.

Techniques 21–23: Big Situps

21. Bring your arms over the head. Inhale and hold your breath.

22. Smoothly raise your arms, lift both legs, touch ankles. Pause.

23. Lower your legs and arms to mat. Then exhale. (Bend both knees if you find it impossible to raise off your mat with legs straight.) Pay attention to this tricky breath pattern. Flow smoothly from 21–23. Repeat 6 times.

Techniques 24–27: Alternate Leg Lifts

24. Come up onto your right elbow. Inhale. Raise your right leg up and reach your left hand up to touch (do not grab on) your right ankle. Pause.

25. Exhaling, lie back down on your mat. Pause.

26. Come up onto your left elbow. Inhaling, raise your left leg and right arm. Repeat 24–26 six times, alternating legs.

27. Cross your ankles (or do a Full Lotus, if comfortable). Bring right elbow to the mat. Left arm is relaxed over head. Try to keep your sitting bones on the mat! Hold in a relaxed manner for 10–30 seconds. Repeat on your opposite side.

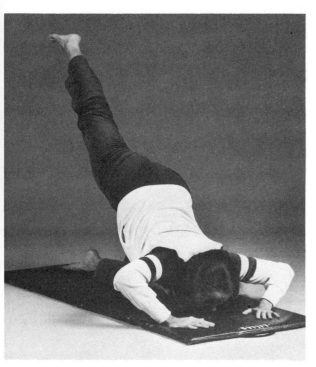

Plank (No. 13-14)

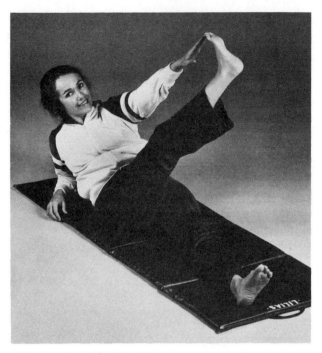

Alternate Leg Lifts (No. 24)

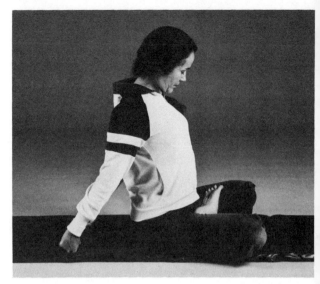

Kundalini Arch (No. 28)

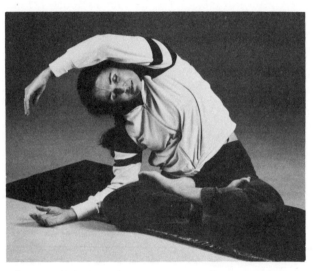

Alternate Side Stretch (No. 27)

Technique 28: *Kundalini Arch*

Sitting with ankles crossed or in Lotus position, make a fist with both hands. Place them on the mat behind you. Sit tall. Inhale, lungs half full. Holding your breath, squeeze shoulder blades together, arching the spine. Then simultaneously tighten your anal muscles and lock your chin to your throat. Hold the breath and chin and anal lock for 10 seconds. Release slowly. Repeat 2 to 3 times.

Lie down. Relax. You deserve it!

MANAGING YOUR TENSIONS AND STRESS

You can manage your own tensions and stress creatively. I suggest you start by rereading this chapter. Then add the following four steps, which are important excerpts from other chapters.

Technique 1

Do the office chair exercises from chapter 15, during your office day. Zero in with exercises on these tension areas: the neck, shoulders, lower back, and abdomen.

Technique 2

Do your "anytime" breathing exercises (Complete Breath) from chapter 4. They will calm you down, increase your energy, help your concentration, and cool disturbing emotional reactions.

Technique 3

Learn how to relax with the relaxation and tension-relieving techniques from chapter 3. You can learn to relax in a chair, standing in a line, or while preparing for bed.

Technique 4

Learn the emotional-stability routine from pages 84–85. Improper breathing habits can increase tension and emotional instability. This routine breaks through that breath pattern and also tones the entire body.

There are only six ways you can move your spinal column—forward, backward, side, right, left, and a twist in both directions. All 845,000 Yoga postures are variations on those movements!

13
Back Talk

THE SPINAL COLUMN

The spinal column is a series of 26 vertebrae that protect your spinal cord. The cord, which is 2 to 3 feet according to height, and an inch wide below the mid-brain, gradually getting smaller, is a network of nerves that services every part of the body.

Each vertebra is cushioned by a disc, a pudding-like substance. Long ligaments support the spine and very small ligaments make up part of each vertebra.

BACKWARD ARCH

The Cobra gently arches the spine backward. This arch opens up and stretches the anterior ligaments or front of the spine. This opening movement increases the flow of blood to the discs, spinal nerve roots, and ligaments. (It is interesting to note that this "front area" is exceedingly difficult to reach with "regular" exercises.)

FORWARD BEND

The opposite, or Forward Bend movement, opens the *back* of the spine, stretches the posterior liga-

ment and root nerves, and gives nourishment to the other side of the discs between the vertebrae.

TWISTING AND SIDE-TO-SIDE MOVEMENTS

Twisting and side-to-side motion promotes spinal flexibility. It keeps space between the vertebrae and maintains proper spinal alignment.

Advanced age, or new injuries, poor posture, poor nutrition, lack of the proper type of exercise, all have negative effects on the spinal column. When the spine becomes stiff, shortened, or "settled," the spaces between the vertebrae are shortened. Little by little, nerves become crowded, thereby increasing possibility of cutting down their energy supply. Pinched spinal nerves may bring on headaches, eye strain, indigestion, and other ailments.

NATURAL CURVES OF THE SPINE

The natural curves of the spine give the entire back resiliency and strength. At birth a baby has only a single curve of the spine. That is the middle

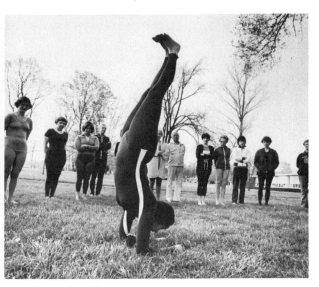
Straight Back Talk

back (thoracic curve). As the baby lies on the stomach in a crib, he or she begins to lift the head, and the curve of the upper neck begins to form. The infant has also spontaneously done its first Yoga posture—the Cobra! The baby soon learns to stand, causing the lower-back (lumbar) curve to form, thus completing the second posture—Standing Pose.

STIFF JOINTS

The spine is also the longest set of articulate joints of the body. All movable joints of the skeletal system are lubricated with synovial fluid. This is the "grease" that enables joints to move in all directions. Some doctors think that improper exercise, combined with a highly acidic diet, produces acid crystals and inorganic calcium-like substances that lodge themselves in the space between the joints and gradually displace the synovial fluid, causing pain and stiffness. The doctors further theorize that the six spinal movements release the toxins from the spine and joints, thereby reducing pain and stiffness.

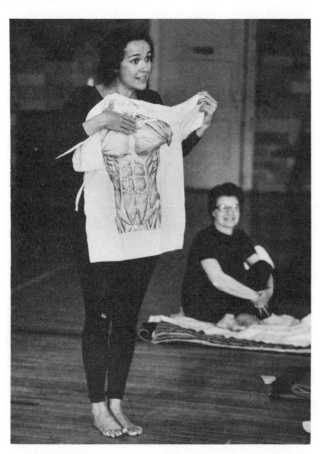

Muscle Memory

MUSCLE MEMORY

Muscles move the body's 206 bones, including the spine. Muscles move bones; bones do not move muscles.

Researchers have found that physical and emotional trauma is registered in muscle. Both physical and mental stress from the past can be worked out and released carefully and slowly, through Yoga exercises and breathing.

Feelings of restlessness, frustration, even anger during a Yoga class are common. If any of these happen to you, keep in mind it's part of the cleansing process. Negative emotions, long locked in the muscles, are finally *leaving* you! (See page 83 for more on depression.)

CIRCULATION

Circulation acts as the transport system of the body, removing toxins and giving nourishment. The squeeze-hold-release action of many Yoga postures stimulates circulation and is another reason why people feel better after a half hour of Yoga.

A CASE HISTORY

As the years go by and the spine is left unattended, the lower back will sway and abdominal muscles will lose their strength and elasticity. Then the serious back problem becomes more than just a possibility.

The abdominal muscle acts as a splint for the spinal column. When the abdominals are weakened through inactivity or childbirth, the lower back must supply almost total support, putting a great strain on an already weak area.

Back problems also arise in tense people. Men and women without channels for their emotional energies tend to collect their tension in weak spots such as the lower back.

Jim Greenwood is 43, married, and the father of 5 children. He has been an architectural engineer for 25 years and sometimes sits bent over a drafting board for 70 to 80 percent of his day.

My working day lasts anywhere between eight and sixteen hours, sometimes six to seven days a week. Before

I noticed I had a weak lower back, I could not go through a full eight-hour day without feeling exhausted. I would stoop to pick up catalogs or lower my head for the drinking fountain and come up dizzy. I ran and walked some, but felt listless and bored about formal exercising.

Then I had a serious fall about five years ago, and my back went out. I realized that lack of exercise had left me with little muscle tone. My doctor explained that the muscular system of my back was not strong enough to hold the vertebrae in place. He also suggested I do a series of back exercises and use some of the tools Yoga could give me.

At first I learned from a book. I lost weight, felt a little better, but there was something missing! I realized once I got into a Yoga class that the thing that was missing was breathing and the body working together.

For a year now I have done one day of my regular Yoga routine, and the next day I work on specific back-talk exercises. It's working!

I'm looking better, and feeling better. And because I now think more positively, I deal more confidently with people on a business and personal level.

EXERCISES FOR THE BACK

You do not have to be a five-star Yogi to do the following exercises. They are very easy and should feel wonderful. Just find 20 or 30 minutes each day and enjoy!

Helpful Hints

If you are now experiencing lower-back discomfort, check with your physician before starting this or any other exercise program.

Take a warm bath to release muscle tension before you start exercises.

Do the exercises instead of sitting when your back aches and feels tired!

Be realistic about your sore back. It's taken more than a few years to let your back get out of shape. It will take more than a few weeks to restore it to normal flexibility and strength.

Learn to distinguish between discomfort and pain. Pain means stop at once and talk to, or see your doctor. Discomfort very likely occurs when you first start these exercises. In a sense, a small amount of muscle discomfort means progress.

Read over the entire exercise before trying it.

Do not rush through any exercise.

Be attentive to the breathing cycles.

Relax between exercises. Read chapter 12, "Creative Stress—Creative Tension." Ponder how this subject might apply to your back soreness.

Try to exercise every other day. But don't feel

guilty and stop entirely if you miss a few days. Start again.

Do not just slide unconsciously through the movements. Be aware of your plan, which exercises follow which, and how long the hold, etc.

Place pillows under your knees if your back bothers you during Relaxation, or relax curled up on your side.

Do the Sponge or Relaxation Pose, chapter 16, after your exercise session. When you are through with your 10-minute Relaxation, turn over onto your left side; curl up into a fetal position and rest; then come into the sitting position.

The First Week

TABLE

The Table is a starting position for many different Asanas. The placement of your hands and knees and spine is important.

Kneel. Lean forward and place both hands on your mat.

Your spine must be in a straight line. The body forms a table.

Look down and check to see that knees are 12 inches apart and directly beneath the hips; and your hands are beneath your shoulders, 12 inches apart. Remember to pull the abdomen up!

CAT ARCH

This is wonderful for the entire spinal column. It is especially designed to relax your lower-back muscles and relieve painful spasms or cramps in the lumbar region.

Place your body in the Table pose.

Exhale. Bring your chin to your throat; round the spine; contract the buttocks muscle.

Inhale. Raise the chin; concave the lower spine as if to bring tail bone up toward the ceiling.

TORSO TWIST

This exercise will gently twist and stretch the muscles of the middle and lower back. In this slow stretch, you will gently ease away your back tensions, and will straighten this important group of muscles that give vital support to your lower back.

Start with Table pose.

Inhale smoothly. Lift your right arm up toward

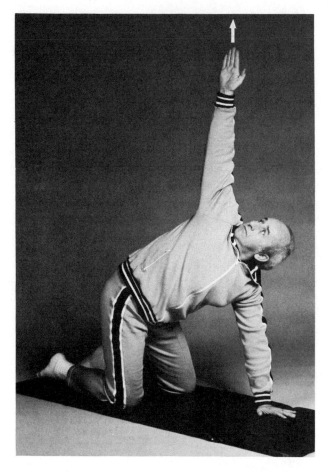

Torso Twist

the ceiling as far as possible. Look up to thumb of your right hand. Hold 3 seconds

Return to Table pose.

Repeat with your left arm.

DOG WAG

This exercise is designed to remove the stiffness and tension from your lower back and restore its suppleness.

Place your body in the Table pose.

Bring your thumbs together.

Exhale. Look around the side of your right arm.

Move your lower back and hip in a *lateral* motion as far to the right as possible. Try and see your right hip as you look around your shoulder. Hold 3 seconds.

Inhale. Go back to Table pose.

Exhale. Move your hip laterally to the left. Look around upper left arm. Hold 3 seconds.

Inhale. Back to Table pose; then, move laterally, side-to-side, much like a dog wags its tail.

Do not rock the hips. The Dog Wag is a slow,

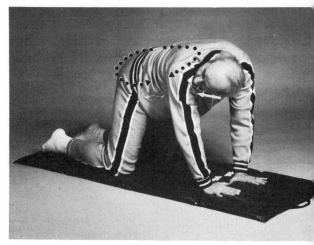

Dog Wag

lateral motion, side to side. As your suppleness increases and tension decreases, this movement will be easier.

Keep trying to see your hip around your shoulder.

MECCA AND POSE OF A CHILD

Place your body in the Table pose.

Keep your hands flat on the floor as you sit on your heels.

Now try to walk forward with your fingertips, while still sitting.

Feel your lower and middle back and shoulders stretch as you reach. This entire movement should make your lower back feel wonderful!

Place your hands, palms up, back alongside the body. Turn your head to the side to rest on mat. This posture is called Pose of a Child. Take a few comfortable breaths and relax deeply.

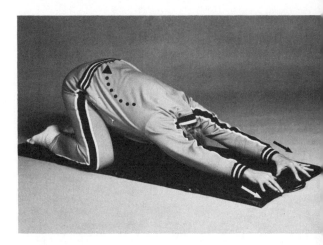

Mecca Pose

Variation

Instead of placing hands alongside the body bend elbows and make your hands into separate fists. Reach around and gently pummel the muscles of your lower back. Do not hit your spinal column, just the muscle on either side. Then relax arms once again.

With knees 2 feet apart rest in Pose of a Child.

The Second Week (Standing or Kneeling)

WAIST TWIST

Relax your arms; bend the elbows.
Twist from waist only, first one side, then the other.
Start at 5 times each side. Work up to 20.

CLENCHED FIST

With arms alongside body, make a fist with both hands.
Bring them to your chest.
Tense your arms and exhaling, pull your shoulder blades together. Release. Inhale; then exhale.
Repeat from 5 up to 20 times.
Do Shoulder Rotations, forward and backward, page 17; and Neck Tilt, page 22.

The Third Week (Standing)

UPPER-BODY TWIST

Stand with feet together, with arms relaxed or bent.
Twist upper torso and hips to the right, then to the left.
Repeat 5 times. Work up to 20.

ROTATING HIPS CLOCKWISE

Stand with feet well apart, arms at the sides.
Rotate hips clockwise.
Repeat 5 times. Work up to 20.

DOOR HANG

This exercise is not a *must*. It's fun to do occasionally when your lower back feels tired.
Clasp your hands firmly on the upper edge of

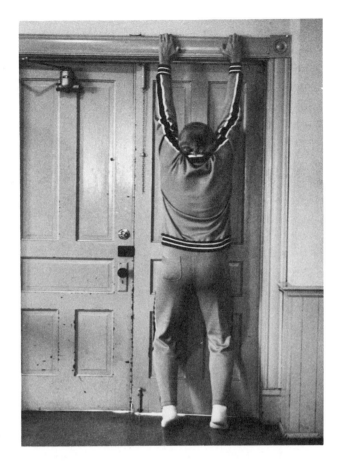

Door Hang

a sturdy door that will not swing closed quickly. Then let your body go limp. Hold, body relaxed for 30 seconds.
Bend your knees and let your body hang limply.
Be sure you feel the weight of your body in your lower body and not just in your arms. You should feel relief in your lower back.
Keep arms strong by tensing them slightly.
Hold for 5 seconds. Repeat 3 times.

The Fourth Week

ARM AND LEG LIFT

A powerful back-extension exercise designed to strengthen the lateral muscles of the lower back as well as those of the buttocks, front and backs of the thighs.
Place your body in the Table pose.
Inhale and *slowly* raise the right leg up toward the ceiling. Raise the chin and look up.
Raise your right arm as high as possible.
Breathe comfortably, as you hold this position 10 seconds.

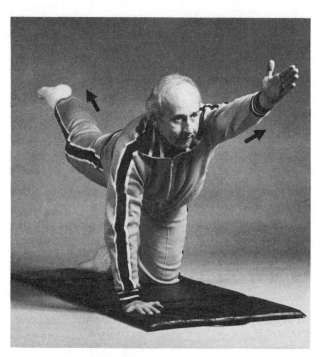

Arm and Leg Lift (Table Pose)

Return to Table.
Repeat on opposite side.
Increase slowly up to 15 seconds.

Variation
Place body in Table pose.
Inhale and slowly raise your right leg up toward ceiling.
Then raise your left arm up as high as possible.
Once you get your balance, keep that lift steady for 10 seconds.
Work up to a hold of 30. Then rest in Mecca pose.

The Fifth Week (On Your Mat)

EASY ROCK-AND-ROLL

Lying on your mat bring your knees to your chest, and clasp your wrists behind your knees.
Now, rock back and forth *just* on your lower back. This should feel good and give a nice massage to this area.
Keep the movement up for 30 to 50 seconds.

PELVIC TILT

The pelvic tilt is mentioned in chapter 5. Go back to the original and read thoroughly the mechanics of this exercise.

HEAD-TO-KNEE POSE

This exercise strengthens as well as soothes a weak lower back. It promotes better circulation to the intestinal tract, helping to eliminate indigestion, gas and cramps.
Lie down on mat.
Do Pelvic Tilt.
Tighten buttock muscle. Bend knees slightly.
Exhale, and press your lower back to floor firmly.
Repeat 3 times.
Inhale, and bring both knees to chest. Raise arms and place hands over lower legs. (If you have knee problems, bring arms behind knees.)
Exhale, and press thighs to chest simultaneously raising head, and bring your head as close as possible to knees.
Hold pose for 10 to 30 seconds. DO NOT HOLD BREATH. Be sure you are breathing comfortably and relaxing your shoulder and facial muscles.
Flex feet while in this hold.
Release. Holding onto legs, lower head to floor. Take 2 slow, even breaths, relaxing face, shoulders and feet.
Bring feet to mat, then straighten your legs to mat.
Repeat 5 times each side. Add one each day, increasing up to 15.

SLANT BOARD

The Slant Board increases spinal flexibility, top and bottom. This gentle motion strengthens and stretches muscles and ligaments attached to the spine and this is helpful in retaining proper alignment of the vertebrae.

Step 1
Lie on your back; keep arms close to your body. Bend both knees. Place feet straight ahead, heels close to seat muscles. Knees are hip distance apart. Inhale through nose. Exhale. Do Pelvic Tilt. Hold 5 seconds. Release. Repeat 3 times.
Contract seat muscle. Flatten lower back to the floor. Slowly raise each vertebra off the floor, starting at base of spine, and working your way between shoulder blades (shoulders and back of head stay on floor). This entire movement should take at least 10 to 15 seconds. Hold 15 seconds. Open eyes. See that knee, hip, and chest form a "slant board." Breathe comfortably through nose.

Step 2
Slowly raise arms over head until back of hands

Lilias, Yoga, and Your Life

touch floor. Inhale deeply. Exhale slowly. Then, lower arms and spine simultaneously down to the floor. (This should take at least 15 seconds to complete.) Breathe comfortably and evenly.

Repeat 3 times.

Straighten both legs. Close eyes.

Take 3 deep breaths. Observe the effect of the exercise both inside and outside of body.

Increase time for this exercise to one minute over a few weeks.

The Sixth Week (On a Footstool)

If you do not own a footstool, improvise one by making a firm 12-inch-high roll using blankets. The point is to raise the pelvis and torso up higher than just a rolled towel or small pillow would allow.

SWAN DIVE

Lying prone place a firm pillow on a footstool. Lie down prone on top of pillow.

Place your arms out to sides as if in a swan dive. Knees are on the floor. Place forehead on floor. Tighten the seat muscle and tilt the pelvis.

Inhale and lift head and chest up.

Squeeze seat muscle even harder! Hold 3 seconds. Exhale and lower forehead to floor.

Repeat 3 times. Work up to 5.

LEG LIFT

Lying prone on stool place elbows on floor. Scoot chest up slightly on footstool if needed.

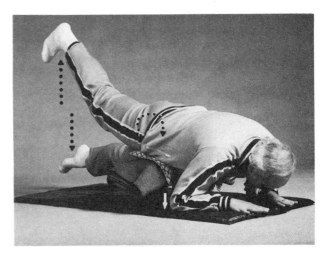
Swimmer's Kick

Tighten the seat muscle *firmly*. Tilt the pelvis.

Inhale and raise both legs up, feet apart. Hold 3 seconds. Exhale and lower.

Repeat 3 to 5 times.

SWIMMER'S KICK

Lying prone over stool, support yourself on your elbows. (Scoot hips forward on stool, if needed.) Be comfortable. Tilt the pelvis.

Stiffen legs. Then kick them up and down in a swimmer's motion.

Kick for 10 to 20 seconds. Rest and repeat.

The Seventh Week

TRUNK LIFT

Lying prone over a stool, hook your feet under a sofa, or desk. Place towel over heels if pressure bothers you.

Clasp hands behind neck, forehead to floor. Tighten the seat and tilt the pelvis.

Inhale and raise your head and chest up high.

Hold 10 to 20 seconds.

Breathing comfortably, lower and repeat 5 to 10 times.

Variation

Repeat above exercise. This time, arms are straight in front.

Hold for 10 seconds. Work up to 20. Increase up to 10 times this number

Relax with Cat Arch and relaxation techniques. Follow routine with hot bath.

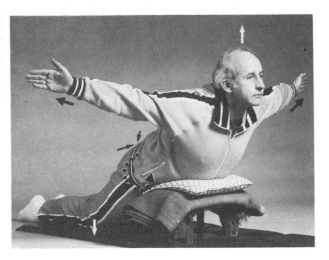
Swan Dive

14

Yoga in Sports

Fitness authorities, as well as athletes all over the world, are discovering that Hatha Yoga stretches and philosophy are excellent for preventing injuries and enhancing the enjoyment of many sports.

Yoga stretches cause muscle groups to contract, lengthen, and relax. The joints attain their full range of motion. Energy flows freely and equally into all parts of the body, and the body achieves proper alignment, making it possible to breathe deeply and fully.

The individual's ability to relax plays a vital part in an athlete's physical and mental health. Physiologically, when a muscle fails to be given time to relax and cool down after a hard workout, it has a tendency to stay tight and shortened. Learning how to relax mentally before or during a game is another challenge that could be a key element in bettering performance. However, most of us do not even know how to relax in daily life, much less during the stress of athletics. Understanding that relaxation is a step-by-step thought process will help you immensely. I suggest you reread chapter 12 "Creative Stress—Creative Tension," where you will find some valuable tools to help you on the court, field, slopes, or track, as well as in your daily life.

Interview with a Surgeon and an Athletic Trainer

Founded in 1975, the University of Cincinnati's Sports Medicine Institute is devoted to multidisciplinary research on the athlete. I interviewed Frank R. Noyes, M.D., an orthopedic surgeon and an associate professor of orthopedic surgery at the University of Cincinnati Medical Center, as well as Robert Mangine, a licensed physical therapist, certified athletic trainer in the National Athletic Trainers Association, and the director of the rehabilitation program at the Sports Medicine Institute.

Mangine: Fifty percent of recreational athletic injuries could have been prevented.

Lilias: What are the components of a good conditioning program that would decrease this percentage?

Mangine: There are 3 components to a good conditioning program. If an athlete intends to play sports, either recreational or organized, in college or high school, she or he has got to be flexible, strong and enduring. If you're not strong, you're going to get hurt as soon as the game starts because the muscles won't fire right and are very susceptible to muscle injury. If you're not flexible, you cannot achieve maximum strength, because you don't allow your joints and muscles to achieve full range of motion, and also you'll be more susceptible to muscular strain, muscular tendon strain, or a tendon rupture. Flexibility is a very, very important part of a conditioning program! Whenever an athlete comes in here, we check him for flexibility, strength and endurance.

Lilias: Let me ask you, Dr. Noyes, from the sports medicine point of view, what does the total athlete mean to you?

Noyes: We've always known that an athlete had to be strong, and so we've always had athletes working on strength exercises, and pushing weights. We've had a whole science of how do you push weights effectively to build strength, i.e., muscle mass. We know that we do it slowly and purposefully; we do it to fatigue muscles so that this increases muscle bulk and strength. We know that muscles can contract very strongly, but to maintain that we have to have endurance—the repetitive firing of muscles such as in long-distance running, swimming—those types of activities.

Then, there's the whole science of muscle enzymes, oxygen consumption, specific training for endurance. Now we have a strong athlete and one who can go for a long period of time. So now we have to add two additional concepts to complete the package of an athlete. One is flexibility. Flexibility is the concept of allowing the joint to go through the full range of motion. A muscle has to contract just at the right time, and we have to let the joint go all the way back to get that stroke-stretch out of that muscle tissue. If you don't and the muscle contracts at the wrong time, it's going to fire at a tremendous burst of force, and it's going to rupture—rupture muscle fibers or a tendon. There'll be swelling, and you're going to have pain and injury.

Another concept, a most important one, is neuromuscular coordination. That's the synthesis of the whole thing. That's where the brain perceives a change in body position and says that you need to fire a muscle right now, or you're going to fall. So first coming up from that reflex arc is, "My ankle is going out," or, "My knee is going out," or, "I'm coming out of a jump, and I've got to be set up just right." This goes all the way to the brain; the brain perceives it and automatically calculates which muscles have to do what and it sends the impulse back down; the muscles contract at the right time. For that muscle to work properly, we have to have the right reflex arc, the right training, coordination, and then the muscle must have the right strength, the right endurance, and the right amount of flexibility. You can't remove one part from the total package concept. As Bob said, in about half the cases I see here the injuries could have been prevented if they'd had this concept of the total package.

Lilias: Do you stress the importance of proper breathing?

Mangine: Probably not as thoroughly as you do in Yoga. We suggest that the athletes do deep breathing during our prescribed exercises, and we try to talk about relaxation.

Lilias: Do you think the average amateur athlete knows how to stretch properly?

Mangine: The average organized athlete does not know how to stretch out! If high school and college athletes with their elaborate training programs don't know how to stretch, how can we expect the average weekend player to know the basic principles of stretching?

Lilias: What do you think about "bouncing?"

Mangine: We believe in holding the body in a steady, quiet, static stretch or at that "edge" that comes just before discomfort. Look at it on a neuromuscular level. Muscles have very strong fibers, two of which are for stretching. If you have a rubber band and you bounce the rubber band back and forth, it's always going to just come right back. These myofibers are like rubber bands. If you stretch them and hold that stretch, the muscle fibers become adapted to that new resting length. As opposed to bouncing up and down, which will cause

the muscle fiber to contract when you finish the stretching exercise.

Lilias: Is that what's called a stretch reflex?

Mangine: Yes. That's what prevents you from getting hurt. If you stretch too far, that little muscle fiber stretches. It is goes too far, it will contract the muscle. As a protective mechanism, there are two components—one is the tendon, and one is in the muscle itself. Both are sensitive to stretch. If you stretch them, they'll stay stretched to the new rested length. As soon as you have a lack of activity, they'll automatically shorten back up. That's why you stretch every day, why a cat stretches every day, to see that these fibers can stretch to a resting length. If you bounce, this shortens them.

Lilias: What causes tennis elbow, or shoulder problems?

Mangine: The number-one cause of tennis elbow is too much activity too soon without prior conditioning and stretching. Weakness in the forearm and arm muscles due to poor conditioning greatly enhances the chance of tennis elbow to develop in the first place.

There are some general dos and don'ts in effective rehabilitation of the arm-shoulder unit that are really a matter of common sense. The major do in any muscle weakness requires at least two or three months of intensive daily exercise for rehabilitation. If the exercises are performed occasionally, there will be little or no benefit. Don'ts are common sense. Exercise should not cause swelling or pain. If this occurs, it often means that there has been too much exercise done *too fast*.

Lilias: Those are also the basic principles of Yoga; go slowly, build up, and play your edge.

How important is it for people over thirty-five to stretch?

Mangine: If you don't stretch, you're going to end up very vulnerable to Achilles tendon ruptures, hamstring ruptures, occasional quad ruptures. These are the three areas that are most affected when there is no stretching.

Lilias: What about men with short, bulky muscles who say they can't stretch?

Mangine: I say they *can* if they dedicate themselves to it. They may have a limit. I am built that way; my muscles are very tight. Even though other therapists here definitely have more of a stretch potential than I do, I can still achieve something by stretching and can thus decrease my chances of injury by stretching.

Lilias: For an amateur athlete interested in Yoga stretches, how many times a week would you suggest doing stretches?

Mangine: We suggest once a day. For sports requiring running we recommend up to twenty to twenty-five minutes of stretching prior to jogging, and five to ten minutes of stretching after their practice session. For golf or tennis, we recommend stretching ten to fifteen minutes. If you do not play any sport, you should still stretch to maintain muscle tone, or else you'll shorten those muscle fibers. So, it's important to stretch each day!

Interview with a Baseball Player

I read in the *Yoga Journal* that the Los Angeles Dodgers used Yoga postures as part of their training, so I went to visit Bill Buhler in Los Angeles at Dodger Stadium, who said:

Let me tell you how it all started. The L.A. Dodger team has been doing what we call static stretches for years, but really they are Yoga postures. We just went into the Yoga books and found positions that would get directly into the areas we needed to stretch out. For example, pitchers find the Plow useful for arms and back; catchers might use the Fish or Bridge for knees, thighs, and groin. Of course, I don't use the Sanskrit

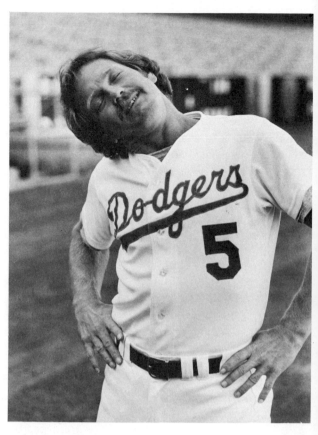

Johnny Oates demonstrates Neck Roll. "I don't go on the field without my twenty minutes of Yoga stretches."

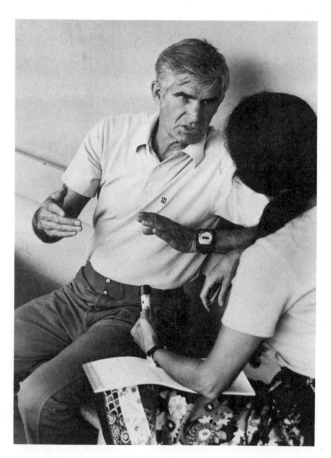

Bill Buhler, trainer of LA Dodgers. "We called them static stretches for years, but they really are Yoga postures."

names, but everything *is* slowed down and nothing done on a cadence.

When I asked him if he had met any resistance either from management or players, his answer was:

Management and Tommy LaSorda have given me terrific support! As far as the players go, we started out with five curious guys, with others watching. The five found it was nothing strange or peculiar, and that it seemed to feel good. Within a few weeks, others joined. Soon we were up to sixty. We concentrated on Yoga stretches in spring training. We all lay out on the grass and spent thirty to forty-five minutes going through different postures, stretches, breathing, and little relaxations. Steve Garvey is much more flexible and has lost inches off the bulk muscles developed from his Michigan State football days, and Johnny Oates says that he doesn't go on the field without doing twenty minutes of his own Yoga routine. He tells me it prepares him both mentally and physically.

Of course, we use it in conjunction with a weights-and-running program. Although I can't say it has cut back on injuries, it has definitely cut back on *recovery* time. When a fellow pulls a hamstring, we'll try stretching it gently. Yoga increases the players' awareness in working with these problems. We make sure all the players do static stretches well before the game because, when they don't, muscles get shorter and therefore more susceptible to pulls and strains.

Interview with a Tennis Pro

I met with Tony Trabert some years back at a tennis workshop while struggling with my backhand. Even though I knew Tony had not officially studied Yoga, I could feel that he was an open and curious man, willing to expand his thinking and push his edges of flexibility physically as well as in his own life. When it came time to write this book, I wanted very much to interview him. We had fun exchanging ideas and exercises.

Most players at the top, as well as amateurs, should do some mild stretch-outs before play. The Davis Cup players, for example, have their own routine. Basically, they are worried about the hamstring and thigh area, also upper arms and shoulders, so they are pretty careful about warming up these areas either on the court or in the locker room. They are also concerned about the lower back, so there usually is some side-to-side and forward movement.

We're all taught to warm up carefully and cool down slowly. I recommend they wear a sweater for warmups until the muscles have become elongated and soft. When the body is sweating and hot after play, I warn that they should take care not to ride home with the air conditioner going full blast or have the arm hanging out the window when they're soaking wet. That is just asking for trouble.

Personally, I jog up to two miles a day with my wife Em. I also do a few stretches each day, but not the traditional Yoga exercises.

I asked him if he wanted to give a few poses a try. Working on just the areas he'd talked about, hamstrings, sides of the body, and upper back and arms. We worked with a towel in the Forward Bend, and used the racket itself in the Over-the-Head Arm Clasp. As you can see from the photos, his natural grace and coordination translated themselves beautifully into these Yoga stretches.

When I left, I kiddingly asked him if he'd keep on working with Yoga stretches. He answered me with a big grin. "I'll try. It felt terrific! In fact better then I expected."

How nice to have an excuse to go back for a visit and a Yoga checkup!

Tony Trabert's natural grace and coordination translates beautifully into Triangle Pose.

Interview with a Long-Distance Runner

The lower half of the runner's body is usually stronger than the upper half.

A simple Yoga routine done each day will balance these effects and add resiliency. Yoga postures are excellent for warmups and cool-downs. They beautifully complement the cardiovascular strength that running promotes.

Craig Virgin is a premier long-distance runner, a Big 10 and NCAA champion at Illinois. And at this writing he holds the U.S. record for the 10,000-meter race with a time of 27:39. He had practiced the Yoga stretches for only 6 weeks before we met. For 22-year-old Craig, these exercises were not that easy, nor were they relaxing; in fact for him they were downright painful. I hope all of you who find these stretches difficult will be inspired by this courageous and determined young man.

Lilias: Do you do any physical exercise other than running? And what are the other parts of your training?

Virgin: One is weight lifting, which for most people would be very light—just a bar with 50 or 60 pounds on it—and I do pushups. Also, I use free weights, dumbbells (the hand-held weights), and lately adding some Yoga static stretches for flexibility.

Lilias: What are some of the physical problems of a long-distance runner

Virgin: You're dealing with a fatigue level. You can get very fatigued, to the point where your resistance is lowered. If you overtrain you can become susceptible not only to illnesses, but also to injuries. Along with fatigue usually comes a certain amount of tightness, stiffness, soreness. Obviously, it seems much worse the first several weeks of your running. But for me, the discomfort comes from the high level of training, which would include about one hundred miles a week, not just running ten to fifteen miles a day, but doing different types of running—hill work, long runs, speed work. The whole key is working and training as hard as you can, yet staying healthy and injury-free. Once you push yourself over the edge, you're susceptible to injuries. So what I'm trying to do is maximize my training and minimize my down-time due to injuries.

Lilias: During training, do you feel any lower-back discomfort?

Virgin: Most of the time I've been pretty healthy. I do have some congenital problems with my back, but I rely on chiropractic checkups three to five times a month as well as applied kinesiology and prescribed physical therapy. My problem the last several years has been an aching lower back, which occasionally goes into spasms. It gets very stiff and tight, especially after a hard race or workout. It's very important for me to have my neck, back and shoulders very relaxed. If I have problems with them, it affects my performance. The whole key to running to your maximum is being as relaxed as possible.

Lilias: How did Hatha Yoga come to be part of your training?

Virgin: I first heard of it three or four years ago when stretching really began to hit the running publications and the runner's consciousness. I did a few mild stretches, using doorways or leaning against trees, etc., before running, but I became more aware of serious stretching when my college coach, Gary Wieneke, talked about it. Until that time I had not been a very serious stretcher. I had achieved a great deal without it; the only question was how much more could I achieve with it? Due to an ambitious business and travel schedule, I have had to put top priority on the time I spend on the aerobic and anaerobic conditioning of my body. But I also try to maximize the time that I put into stretching. Helen Esser, flexibility specialist at the Olympic Camp in Colorado Springs, is the one who introduced me to Yoga.

Lilias: Do you find it easy to stretch?

Virgin: Frankly, right now I don't find it that enjoyable. I'm coping so hard with strong and short muscles and ligaments, that I'm fighting each exercise and feel exhausted when through. At this point it is something that I have to discipline myself to do. It's hard for me to see direct and immediate results from the stretch and how it will affect my performance. Maybe it's because I haven't broken through that initial barrier, like the first two or three weeks in running. There is not that dramatic increase in performance that you can see short-term in running. Yet, in six weeks, I *can* see some improvement with Helen's measuring!

Lilias: The before-and-after measurement that Helen Esser took on you is very encouraging!

Virgin: Yes. It seems that I improved groin-and-thigh-muscle stretches by half an inch. I practiced only on an average of five or six sessions a week, for about fifteen or twenty minutes. Wonder if I could have done a little bit more, and maybe we'd have seen more dramatic results.

Lilias: As you began to work with your breathing with the stretching, what did you notice?

Virgin: I think that was responsible for thirty percent of my improvement

Lilias: What do you hope the increased flexibility will do for your future career in running?

Virgin: That I could go through hard workouts with fewer side effects, less stiffness. In other words, I think it will help me to train just a little bit harder, day after day. I think that looking at the form and technique as such might lengthen my stride without an appreciable amount of effort. Obviously, the more ground you can cover with your stride, the faster you can go with the same amount of energy. To be able to kick at the end of a long-distance race, to withstand the fatigue, requires relaxation. It also requires having it together within your body and mind. It's a delicate balance.

Lilias: You've been using the Yoga stretches to cool down?

Virgin: Finding the time for everything is so hard, as I hold down a regular job during the day. After the evening run, or two or three hours later, I sit in my bedroom, with the music on to make it more pleasant, and practice some of the exercises, breathing, and relaxation. Then I fall into bed. Believe me, I have no trouble sleeping!

Interview with a Yoga Author and Teacher

Helen Esser's flexibility programs are used by coaches and athletes throughout the country. She is the author of two college text books on Hatha Yoga and teaches Yoga at St. Louis Community College at Florissant Valley in St. Louis, Missouri.

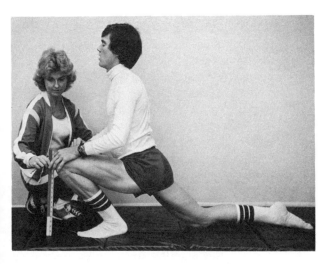

Craig Virgin demonstrates the Forward Lunge. Helen Esser measures for increased flexibility.

She is also on the staff of the U.S. Olympic Development Clinic.

When I asked her about the flexibility-testing procedure, she responded, "All athletes like to see results! If you have the means of testing flexibility, they can see the data, in black and white, that they have improved. I recommend that athletes take the flexibility test every two weeks, making sure to record measurements so they can see progress. Also, if you have the facilities, it's interesting to videotape the students at the beginning of the semester and then three months later. It's an eye opener, and it's exciting to *see* the results on tape! Everyone improves not only in the flexibility test but in their chosen sport as well."

Helen Esser's Flexibility Test uses two measurement devices, a yardstick and clothespin. A clothespin placed on a yardstick enables a more accurate reading while testing flexibility in the Dog stretch and the Bridge, because of the right-angle protrusion of the clothespin.

FORWARD LUNGE

Measure is taken from the upper point where yardstick comes away from the knee. (Photo above.)

DOG STRETCH

Measure the distance between the heel of the shoe and the ground.

Measure the distance from the ground to the head by sliding the clothespin up the yardstick to the head.

BRIDGE

Measure from the middle of the thigh (top of quadriceps) from the ground, using yardstick and clothespin.

Craig Virgin varies this stretch by looping a belt around his ankles.

Interview with Football Players

Before interviewing some of the Cincinnati Bengals, I had a stereotyped view of a football player being a one-dimensional type of man with lots of muscle. What I found was entirely different from what I had expected.

Bengal assistant coach in charge of strength training, Kim Wood, started off by saying, "Yoga stretches should not be looked upon as a fad, but something to be integrated naturally into one's individual routine in preparation for regular practice. These days we are working with the total athlete. Intensive weight training, running, along with stretching all equals balance. Health attitudes and habits should be *continued* in the home as well as on the field, twelve months a year!"

Kim then introduced me to 6'6" Pat McInally, a Harvard graduate, punter, and wide receiver for the Cincinnati Bengals. Pat had won the 1978 punting championship in the National Football League (with a 43.1 average). He commented:

I've come a long way! A year and a half ago I couldn't touch my toes. And that is rather ridiculous for a punter!

I became especially fed up with my stiffness after I noticed that another 6'4" punter was not only kicking the ball farther, but also raising his foot above his head. I figured that if he could get that sort of leverage with his flexibility and his height, just think what I could do with mine.

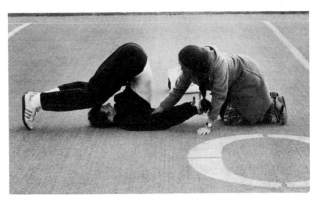

"The problem with most football players is they approach their training as a football player, not as a total athlete." Pat McInally.

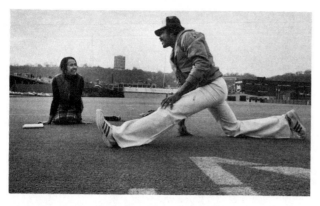

"You bet I have to be careful about stretching out!"—
Isaac Curtis

The problem with most football players is that they approach their training to be only a football player, not a *total athlete*. I decided that along with lifting weights, I would prepare myself to be the best athlete I could be. I began to play two-man volleyball in the sand, as well as taking an intensive stretching program, medically supervised by doctors in Los Angeles. It's paid off. My entire body feels well and in balance, and I'm sending the ball farther than ever. Just think, I spent four years at Harvard without doing one stretching exercise!

Next I chatted briefly with Isaac Curtis, wide runner for the Cincinnati Bengals. He was recovering from a thigh injury.

I'm a runner also. You bet I have to be careful about stretching out! I have my own personal program, just right for me and my body. I've adapted some of the static stretches although I've never called them Yoga, and I use them to warm up before my regular routine. They give me a complete range of motion. Also, I do use the Yoga way of slowly playing around the edge of an injured muscle. This doesn't make it heal faster, but it does help to keep the muscles in and around the area toned and ready for use when I'm ready for my next intensive practice.

How wonderful that the ancient concepts and art of Yoga are being used in such a modern way.

Twelve Helpful Hints for Yoga in Sports

1. Do the postures and stretch series each day as part of warming up or cooling down.
2. Perform each exercise slowly and mindfully.
3. Do not stretch by bouncing up and down. This invokes the stretching reflex, which is exactly *opposite* to the desired slow, controlled stretching of Hatha Yoga.
4. Work your stiffer side first; then hold the position twice as long as the more flexible side.

Without thinking, you will tend to stretch the easier leg first; then work with the stiffer side. Observing the difference, it is easy to feel discouraged and not stay as long in the stretch. Working the stiffer side first will lessen the comparison. Holding it longer regains all-over body balance.

5. Hold each posture 10 seconds; increase that time as you progress. As you hold the Asana, visualize yourself in the perfection of the posture.
6. Release the poses with control and awareness.
7. Coordinate your breathing with your body movements.
8. Think of this practice time as pleasure and adventure, *not* as rigid discipline.
9. Play the edge of your stretches. Playing the edge is moving close to the edge of discomfort, then working with the edge, not going through it. Do not strain! No pain-no gain is an out-of-date, old-fashioned philosophy! This point cannot be overemphasized. Stretching should feel good! If you feel pain, you are overextending.
10. Catch your mind wandering to business, a grocery list, whatever, and bring it back to your pose. This will help strengthen the necessary concentration.
11. When you have an injury that needs rest and healing, carefully stretch muscles *around* the injury. It will help you keep well-conditioned during this recuperative time.
12. Set aside 20 to 25 minutes for slow stretches before you go out onto the track, court, slope, golf course, or playing field.

BACK OF THE LEG WALL STRETCH

Sit sideways to the wall. Then turn and lie down with tailbone close to wall and heels on wall.

Legs are straight and together and kneecaps pulled up. (Optional.) Place rope around balls of feet. Gently pull feet flat.

Rest and hold 30 seconds to 1 minute.

LEGS IN WALL V

Lie down and place your seat close to wall. Then spread your legs apart in a V. Try to keep inner knee close to wall. Massage the inner muscles and ligaments of your thigh.

Rest comfortably. Let gravity pull legs down. Relax your feet.

Rest and hold 30 seconds to 1 minute.

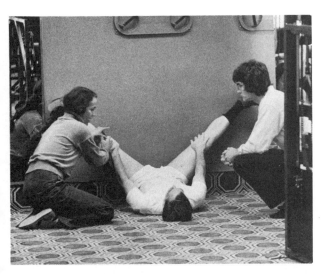

Legs in "V" Off the Wall exercises

WALL GROIN STRETCH

Sit with buttocks as close to a wall as possible.

Bend knees and place soles of the feet together close to the groin.

Place hands on knees and apply gentle pressure to the knee.

Rest and hold 20 seconds to one minute.

WALL LEAN FOR RELAXATION

Stand and place buttocks against a wall. Heels should be 6 inches away from the wall.

Lean all the way forward and go totally limp.

Hold for a half minute.

Breathe comfortably and come up slowly.

FORWARD LUNGE

Kneel on the floor or ground. Stretch your right foot straight in front of you. (Thigh and calf form a right angle.)

Lock your fingers together. Place your palms on your right thigh.

Exhale and project your right knee straight forward beyond your toes keeping your right heel on the ground.

Inhale and breathe deeply. Think *tall,* lift your sternum. Play the edge of the left thigh; stretch. Hold up to 30 seconds.

Release slowly and repeat on the other leg.

As you inhale, you hold the stretch. On the exhalation, relax your muscles and try to move deeper into the stretch, even if it is only a fraction of an inch. This is playing your edge.

FISH

Sit on your knees and heels; let your muscles stretch out. Toes turned under.

Then flatten your feet, instep on the ground or mat. Open the knees and feet 12 inches (hip distance), still sitting on your heels. Lean back and place the elbows on the ground. Hold for 30 seconds. Relax the thigh and groin muscles again.

Proceed only if knees are comfortably on the ground and you are not straining!

Sitting on your heels, bring your weight on the elbows, arch the spine, and roll your head back. Place your head on the ground.

Inhale deeply. Exhale slowly. Hold firmly onto the ankles. This will help you get good spinal lever-

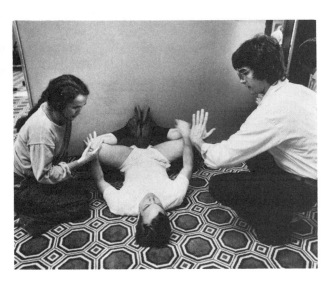

Wall Groin Stretch

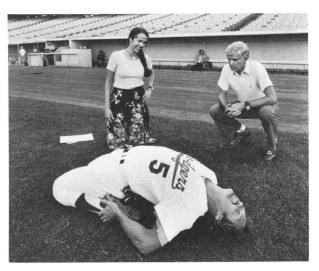

Fish à la Johnny Oates

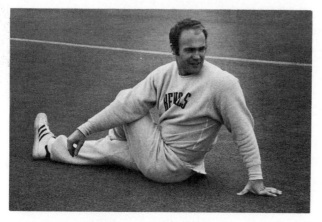

Trainer Kim Wood in Spinal Twist

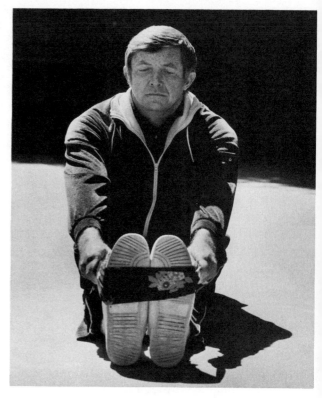

Tony Trabert demonstrates Forward Bend with Towel

age. Hold pose 30 seconds. Do not twist coming up.

Place your hands on the ground, lift the head, push down, then sit up.

Rest in the Star (chapter 7) for 30 seconds.

SPINAL TWIST

Sit on the ground (or mat) with your legs straight out in front of you. Bend the left knee and place your hands on left ankle, then bring your left foot over the right leg. Left foot flat on the ground.

Turn both shoulders to the left; then place the right elbow against your left thigh.

Raise the left arm up and back, placing the hand close to the left buttock.

Inhale deeply. Then exhaling, start to turn each body part individually to the left. Turn the navel to the left rib cage. Pull left shoulder back and *in*, then chin, nose, eyes to your left.

Hold and sit tall, sternum up. Breathe shallowly. Entire movement should take 15 to 20 seconds. Then reverse the processes slowly.

Repeat on the right side.

FORWARD BEND WITH TOWEL

Place your legs directly out in front of you with kneecaps pulled up. Loop a towel behind the ball of one foot.

Inhale, then exhaling, stretch forward, pulling gently on towel (or hands on ankles). Relax the neck. Hold in this position breathing gently for 30 seconds to 1 minute.

Repeat breath pattern and forward movement once again with other foot. Inhale, then, exhaling, rotate your hips, trying to bring your navel toward the thighs. Play the edge of this Forward Bend.

OVER THE HEAD ARM CLASP

Frees the stiffness in armpits. Good warmup for all racket sports, plus pitching and throwing. Releases tension in shoulders and reduces dowager's hump. Relieves stiff arthritic shoulders.

Sit or stand with your spine straight. Raise your right hand and bring it over your head. Bend your elbow and reach down your back as if to scratch your spine. Have a towel within reach.

Bring your left hand up and grab your right elbow. Inhale, then exhale and pull your right elbow in toward the center of your head. Your head is up straight. Your right hand now is lowered down the center of your spine. Release your elbow. This time clasping your towel, reach down your back. The towel is now dangling down your spine.

Bring your left hand down and around and reach up to clasp your towel.

Now pull down on the towel with your left hand. Hold. Then pull up on the towel with your right.

Repeat 3 times with each arm.

As you become more limber, there is no need to use a towel.

Continue.

Bring your left hand down, around, and back within the grasp of your right hand.

Now pull down with your left hand and hold;

Lilias, Yoga, and Your Life

then pull up with your right hand. As you become more limber, take two more breaths and pull your right upper arm and elbow away from your head. Repeat entire procedure with your left hand.

OSTRICH

It's fun to try!

Terrific spine stretch.

Paves the way for inverted postures.

Good warmup stretch for sports that require kicking, such as soccer and football. Also warmup for the Plow, Shoulderstand, and Headstand.

Should not be attempted until the Rock-and-Roll series is comfortable and time has been spent in strengthening the cervical curve of the upper neck with Neck Ups from page 21.

Technique 1

Sit on the floor. Knees are bent. Clasp your hands behind your knees.

Inhale and push with your feet. Roll back until your knees are on your forehead. Separate your knees, resting them on either side of ears and shoulders.

Exhale and lift the spine. Tilt your body toward your chin; lower your knees closer to the floor. Do not force.

Grasp hold of the instep of your right foot with both hands. Push your right knee into your shoulder.

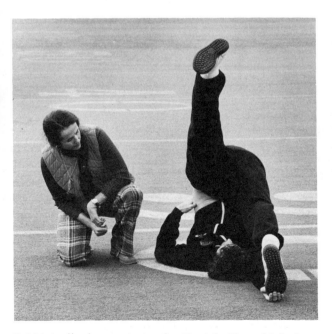

Pat McInally demonstrates the Ostrich. "Just think, four years at Harvard without one stretching exercise."

Your knee is next to the floor.

Inhale and raise the right leg up, right heel to the ceiling; right leg is straight.

Exhale, lowering right leg to the floor in the starting position. Repeat, raising the opposite leg.

Technique 2

After you have limbered up, bring both knees to rest flat on the floor, close to your shoulder.

Bring both forearms to the backs of your knees. Work your fingers between your knees and head. Palms cup both ears. (Note photo.)

Take 3 to 5 normal breaths, or rest until you are ready to come out of the pose. Release your arms and slowly roll down, a vertebra at a time.

Helpful Hints

Relax in the pose.

Do not collapse your chest. Keep a lift within your spine so you can breathe easily.

Work your arms and hands into position. Knees will lower and give you balance.

BRIDGE

Because this posture is so easily done, it is also easy to do incorrectly! The lower curve of the spine (lumbar curve) is made up of five large vertebrae. When you are at the top of the Bridge (note photo), it is simple to painfully squeeze those vertebrae and not leave the space necessary for a healthy, strong lower back. Many months of practice with this type of unconscious pressure while in the posture will *cause* lower-back discomfort rather than remove it.

The remedy is simple. Do the Pelvic Tilt (from the chapter on Building Blocks). Then, think *up* with your hip bones, and imagine your breastbone going toward your chin. This up motion, combined with a Shoulder Rotation, will keep the healthy freedom and space needed within the lumbar and sacral area of the spine.

The Bridge limbers up the spine, makes it more flexible through toning the central nervous system, tightens and forms the seat, reduces midriff fat, and strengthens the wrists. Excellent groin and thigh stretch.

Lie on your back, placing the hands alongside the body. Bend the knees as you bring the heels as close as possible to the seat muscles; knees are hip distance apart, toes forward. Do the Pelvic Tilt. Contract your seat muscles. Inhale; then, exhaling, press the abdomen and the arch of the spine back firmly down toward the floor.

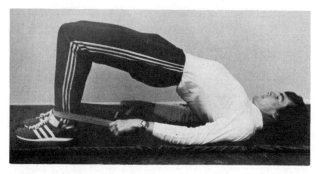

Here Craig Virgin demonstrates the Bridge. He works with his stiffness by placing a belt around his ankles.

Slowly, to the count of 15, (one second one, two seconds two, etc.) feel each vertebra separately as they roll off the ground or mat, starting with the tailbone (coccyx) on up to the vertebrae between the shoulder blades. When you reach the top of the pose, open your eyes and correct the front hip-to-chest angle of your body.

Now lift off the heels to the balls of your feet; tilt the pelvis and think *up* with the hips! Keep that *up* feeling by squeezing and firmly contracting the buttocks muscles, and trying to make the pelvis almost flat. Hold the position 5 to 10 seconds. Then, slowly come down, exhaling to the count of 10 and smoothly lowering the spine to the floor.

STANDING LUNGE WITH CHAIR

I suggest you practice your Lunge for two weeks before attempting the Standing Lunge with Chair. You can get the feel of this pose even in the beginning stages with the ankles, hip sockets, thighs, and legs weak and stiff.

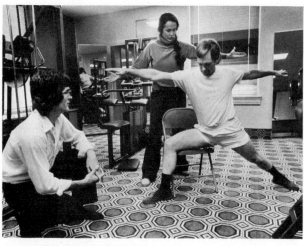

Forward Lunge with Chair

Place your right thigh on the edge of the chair and your right foot on the floor. Look down and adjust your thigh, knee and foot position. Your knee is to be directly over your ankle, forming a right angle to the floor. Your thigh and hip bones are parallel to the floor line.

Then look down and adjust your back anchor leg. Your heel is on the floor, toes turned inward slightly. The weight is on the outer rim of your left back leg. Knee is straight.

Place your weight on your feet; your right thigh rests *lightly* on your chair. You are conscious of *not* having that right knee wander off course! Arms in T position. Think *up* with the sternum and the top of your head. Hold 5 to 10 seconds. Release.

Sit on chair and reverse legs. Repeat entire procedure.

Do not lean back in your chair. Your thigh is balanced comfortably on the front edge.

STEP-UP FOR STRENGTHENING MUSCLES AROUND KNEE

Stand at the bottom of the stairs, both feet together. Place your right foot one step above. Stand tall. Straighten your knee to return the left foot to the floor. Do this up-down motion 10 to 20 times standing as tall as possible. Use the wall banister for balance. Then change legs.

As you get stronger, stretch the leg that is not being worked on out to your side.

PICKING UP MARBLES

For foot flexibility, pick up marbles with your toes. Carry the marbles with toes and drop them into a dish.

HEEL WALK

Stand on your heels to the count of 10, using the wall as support. As you feel stronger, stand on one heel. In a few weeks, try walking on your heels until you are fatigued.

PICKING APPLES

In a standing position raise arms over head and start reaching and stretching upward, alternating with arms. Reach 10 times each side.

NECK ROLL

Sit tall and drop your chin to your throat. Make believe your chin is a pendulum and swing your chin slowly from side to side.

Inhale and make a half circle to the right with your head. Bring your ear toward your right shoulder; then drop your head back.

Exhale, making a half circle with your head to the left. Keep your shoulders straight throughout this movement.

Repeat this Neck Roll 3 times in each direction.

MOON SALUTATION II

All major muscles are stretched in this 10-part series. Torso muscles receive concave, convex, rotation, and lateral flexion.

Stand with your feet approximately 3½ to 4 feet apart. Turn your right foot at a 90-degree angle, rotating your left foot slightly inward toward the center.

1. Place arms in the T position. Exhaling, slide the arms laterally to the right, keeping shoulders parallel to an imaginary wall behind you. Pull kneecaps up. Right hip is rotated back toward wall. This torso position is kept for the next three stretches.
2. Inhaling, take hold of right ankle with right hand. Stretch left hand up toward ceiling, rotating top of your left shoulder and hip back to touch an imaginary wall. Look to thumb of left hand.
3. Exhaling, stretch your left arm straight out to the side. Upper arm should be close to left ear.
4. Inhaling, bend right leg, thigh, and calf to form right angle. Your knee is directly above the ankle. While keeping bent knee projected to the side, place the right hand next to the outside of your right foot. Stretch the left arm up diagonally. Keep rotating ribs and shoulders back to imaginary wall.
5. Exhaling, turn and face your bent leg; then place hands on either side of foot. Project right knee beyond the toes, but keep your right heel on ground. Relax the front thigh muscles of left leg.
6. Inhale. Lock your fingers together and place them on right thigh. Tighten buttocks and arch back. Extend line of navel to sternum. Exhale as you come out of pose.
7. Inhale. Place right hand on right knee, left hand on left thigh. Exhaling, twist, looking

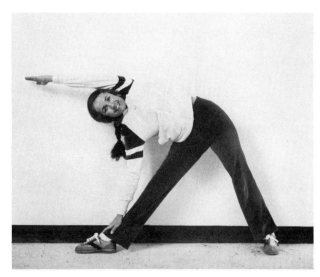

Moon Salutation (3)

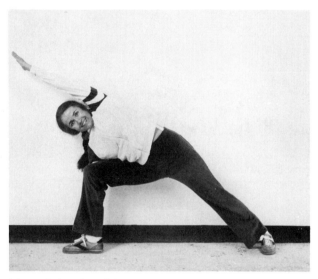

Moon Salutation (4)

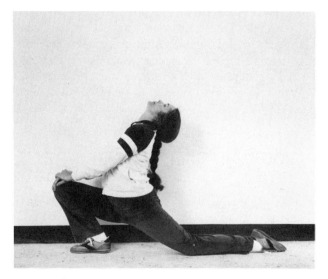

Moon Salutation (6)

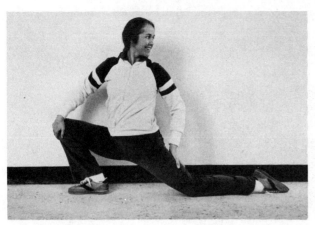

Moon Salutation (7)

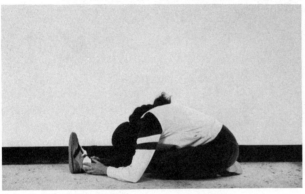

Moon Salutation (9-10)

over your left shoulder. Keep bent knee directly over your foot. See that both legs are stretched into one straight line.

8. Exhale. Turn your torso back to center and place ribs on right thigh and hands on ground on either side of foot.

9. Inhale. Keeping your feet in place, start to sit back on left heel.

10. Exhale. Lower ribs and forehead toward your right leg with hands grasping ankles. You now are sitting on your left heel. Now backtrack your steps in reverse order, going from numbers 10 to 1. Repeat procedure on other side.

PROGRAM FOR THE TOTAL ATHLETE

BODY PART	POSTURE
Complete Body	Moon Salutation
	Sun Salutation
Toes	Picking up Marbles
Foot	Step-up
Ankle and Arches, Heels, Calves	Step-up and Heel Walk
Hip, and foot flexibility	Rock-a-Baby
Inner-thigh muscle and ligament	Legs in Wall V
Groin	Groin Stretch on Wall
	Bridge
	Abdominal Lift
	Forward Lunge
Lower Back	Nose-to-Knee Pose
	Pelvic Tilt
	Bridge
	Dog
	Forward Bend
	Plow
	All back exercises
	Wall Lean
Achilles tendon, hamstrings	Dog Stretch
	Forward Bend with Towel
	Forward Lunge
	Heel Walk
	Hamstring Stretch
	Triangle
	Ostrich
Abdominal muscles	Bridge
	Plow
	Fish
	Abdominal Lift
Knees	Bridge
	Forward Lunge
	Rock-a-Baby
	Fish variations
	Triangle
	Step Up
Sides	Triangle
	Over-the-Head Arm Clasp
Spine	Rock and Roll
	Simple Twist
	Plow
	Forward Bend
	Fish
	Ostrich
Arms and elbows, upper torso	Chest Expander
	All shoulder work
	Over-the-Head Arm Clasp
	Picking Apples
	Triangle
Lungs and respiratory system	Fish
	Breathing exercises
	All shoulder work
	Chest Expander

Lilias, Yoga, and Your Life

Neck	Neck Roll
	Neck Up
	Shoulder Rolls
	Neck Tilt
Relaxation	5-minute Sponge

WEEKLY FLEXIBILITY PROGRAM FOR THE TOTAL ATHLETE

Add this six-week flexibility program to your own practice schedule and observe your improved performance.

All the following exercises can be done wearing sneakers, warmup suits, or shorts. They can be done sitting on your mat at home or outside on the ground. Use them for warming up or cooling down.

The First Week

Standing Hip Rotation and Concave Spine Elongation
Pelvic Tilt
All shoulder work
Step Up
Picking Apples
Over-the-Head Arm Clasp
Picking Up Marbles
All off-the-wall exercises
Dragon Breath
Neck Up and Neck Tilt
Sitback (with arm variations)
Forehead-to-Knee Pose
Rock-and-Roll
Single-Leg Raise with Belt
Rest briefly in Sponge; take 3 Complete Breaths
Double-Heel Descent
Bridge with Shoulder Rotation
Dog Stretch
Pose of a Child; rest 30 seconds
Frog
Vise
Flounder
Star
3 to 6 Complete Breaths
5-minute Sponge relaxation
Read chapter 12, "Creative Stress—Creative Tension"
Read chapter 3, "Creative Relaxation—Your First Yoga Lesson"
Read chapter 13, "Back Talk"

Second Week

Add:
Pendulum Leg Swing
Knees Side-to-Side
Space Walk
The Windmill
Rest in Sponge; take 3 Complete Breaths
Dog Wag
Cat Arch
Twist
Forward Bend with Towel
Hip Rock
6 Complete Breaths
Sponge—3 minutes

Third Week

Add:
Arm and Leg Lift 1 and 2
Slant Board
Forehead-to-Knee Pose
Lunge with Chair
Triangle
Cooling Breath
6 Complete Breaths
Sponge—3 minutes

Fourth Week

Add:
Rest in Sponge; take 3 Complete Breaths
Plow with Chair
Ostrich
Chest Expander
Abdominal Lift
Cleansing Breath
3-minute Sponge

Fifth Week

Add:
Moon Salutation
Take 3–6 Complete Breaths in Sponge
Rest in Sponge 3–5 minutes.

Sixth Week

Add:
Sun Salutation
Take 3–6 Complete Breaths in Sponge
Rest in Sponge 3–5 minutes

YOGA FOR HOCKEY, SOCCER, FOOTBALL, AND LACROSSE

Week One, "Back Talk," p. 89
Weeks Six and Seven, "Back Talk"
All shoulder work exercises
Stretch and Yawn
Complete Breath
Chest Expander, work up to arm movement
Crossed Ankle Rock and Roll
Sitbacks with Arms
All off-the-wall exercises
Forehead-to-Knee Pose
Intermediate Leg Stretch
Maltese Cross
Double-Heel Descent
Plank
Mecca Pose
Vise
Frog
Dancer's Pose
Easy Twist
Forward Bend with Tie
Rock-a-Baby
Dolphin
Moon Salutation
Spinal Warmups
Locust Warmups
Relaxation for 3 to 5 minutes

YOGA FOR BASEBALL, TRACK AND FIELD, AND WRESTLING

Week One, "Back Talk"
Weeks Six and Seven, "Back Talk"
All shoulder work exercises
Yawn and Stretches
Complete Breath
Lemon Squeeze
Bridge with Shoulder Rotation
Neck Tilt
Triangle
Standing Side Stretch
Standing Half-Moon
Dog
Intermediate Leg Raise
All off-the-wall exercises
Sitback with Arms
All Rock-and-Rolls
Sky Diver
Lunge with Chair

Forward Bend with Towel
Plow
Half-Candle
Fist
Vise
Frog
Star
Plank
Inclined Plane with variations
Moon Salutation
Hip Rock
Sponge, 3–5 minutes

YOGA FOR GOLF

Torso Twist
Dog Wag
Cat Stretch
Mecca Pose
Stretch and Yawn
Tense and Hold
Waist Twist
All shoulder work exercises
Lemon Squeeze
Sitback
Chest Expander (with arm variations)
Standing Half-Moon
Rag Doll
Standing or Sitting Foot Flaps
Neck Tilt
Over-the-Head Arm Clasp
Picking Apples
Pendulum Leg Swing
Standing Forehead to Knee
Wall Lean
Bridge with Shoulder Rotation
All Rock-and-Rolls
Knees Side-to-Side
Cobra Warmups
One Leg Forward Bend with Belt
Pushups 1, 2, and 3
Spinal Twist
Complete Breath
Relaxation

YOGA FOR SKIING

Complete Breath
All shoulder work exercises
Off-the-wall exercises

Week One,"Back Talk"
Hydrant
Elongation of Spine—Building Blocks
Chest Expander, Steps 1, 2, and 3
Forehead to Knee Pose
Weeks Six and Seven, "Back Talk"
Dog Stretch
Rock-and-Roll
Lunge Warmup
All off-the-wall exercises
Rag Doll
Advanced Leg Stretch
Moon Salutation
Dancer's Pose
Bridge with Shoulder Rotation
Drawbridge
Frog
Maltese Cross
Space Walk
Pendulum Leg Swing
Crocodile
Double-Heel Descent
Advanced Forward Bend
Plow
Shoulderstand
Fish
Vise
Flounder
Lunge Warmup
All standing poses
Rock-a-Baby
Mecca Pose
Relaxation, 3–5 minutes

Triangle
Intermediate Leg Stretches
Spider
Sitbacks with Arm Variation
Neck Tilt
Neck Roll
Foot Flaps
Spinal Twist
Camel
All Rock-and-Rolls
Bridge with Shoulder Rotation
Drawbridge
Half-Shoulderstand
Fish
Forward Bend with Towel
Inclined Plane
Plank
Lunge Warmups
Any standing poses
Complete Breath
Relaxation, 3–5 minutes

YOGA FOR TENNIS

Pelvic Tilt
All shoulder work exercises
Stretch and Yawn
"Back Talk" exercises
Dog Wag
Cat Arch
Hydrant
Swan Dive
Trunk Lifts
All off-the-wall Exercises
Leg Raises with Tie
Chest Expander
Over-the-Head Arm Clasp
Lemon Squeeze
Standing Side Stretch
Standing Half-Moon

15

Sitting Fit

My interest in Yoga exercises adapted for chair-sitters started many years ago. I'd been teaching for one year, and a student of mine asked me to do my very first lecture-demonstration for her group. I remember driving over in the car, preparing my talk in my head, thinking of all the terrific postures I would show them and all the benefits I had received and could share.

I walked into the meeting room, and what I saw jolted me. The entire room was filled with men and women in wheelchairs. Her "group" was made up of out-patients from the local hospital. Here were people with every kind of problem imaginable, all waiting for my Yoga demonstration.

The spirit has moved through my life many times. This was one of those moments. Life once again held the mirror up for me to take a good look at myself. What I saw wasn't very pretty. I saw my own overinflated ego and pride. Yet at the same moment, I felt a flow of love for these men and women and a surge of inspiration to help those who are bound to sitting most of their lives.

With this inspiration, I guided them through some spontaneously created Yoga exercises they could do in their chairs. By the end of the hour, we all were communicating through smiling faces, pink cheeks, friendly touches, and laughter.

You needn't be bound to a wheelchair to benefit from the exercises in this chapter. Perhaps you are an office worker or a professional who spends much of your working day in a chair. Or perhaps because of a temporary injury, you must sit more than you've been used to. There is no reason why you cannot exercise all 600 muscles of the body while sitting in your chair, and there are many good reasons to exercise them whenever you can. Sitting for lengthy periods of time without moving can slow your circulation and make you feel grumpy, sluggish, and tired. When you are tired, you don't realize that your level of work and concentration of thought are deteriorating.

Exercise can restore energy not only by stimulating circulation but also by relaxing muscles that have been unnecessarily strained while sitting. For example, the business executive who makes phone calls with a tightened fist and clenched teeth, or the secretary who types all day with hunched shoulders, will both feel exceptionally tired at the end of the day.

Improper posture caused by a badly constructed office chair can also sap energy. Be particular about the chair you sit in from 9:00 to 5:00! People sit in chairs; jobs do not! Insist on a chair that does not block off leg circulation; one that has a flat, wide, padded seat, and does not hit you behind the knees. The chair should support your lower back well with a "bun" of firm padding to cushion the pelvis and hold your back erect, thus taking strain off the lumbar curve of the spine. Even if you have a properly constructed chair, prolonged sitting may cause you to slump, putting undue stress on some of your muscles.

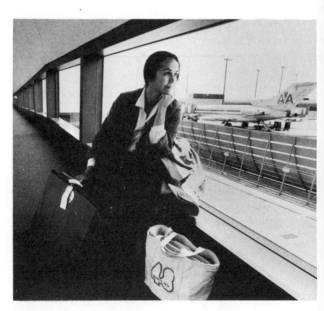

"Have Leotard, Will Travel"

Except for the Tree, which is included here because it, too, fits so easily into an office-exercise program, all of the following exercises adapted from Yoga can be done sitting in a chair, whether it be an office chair, wheelchair, airline seat, or the side of your bed. Before you start this easy 15-to-20-minute Exercise-in-a-Chair Program, loosen your collar, tie, and belt, if possible. Sit straight against the back of your chair (unless asked otherwise). Take off your glasses and place your hands comfortably in your lap. Remember to take a Complete Breath between each exercise and to observe how each movement feels within the muscles. The exercises need not be done all at once; some can be done while talking on the phone or even while working.

I suggest that you read chapter 3, "Creative Relaxation—Your First Yoga Lesson" and chapter 12, "Creative Stress—Creative Tension." They will give you more of an in-depth understanding of how to use the principles of relaxation in your daily life.

EXERCISES ON A PLANE

Some of these exercises can be done on a plane unobtrusively and may help you relax and avoid travel ills, such as digestive problems and constipation.

At check-in time on a long flight get an aisle seat so you can get up and walk. When you walk, stretch out your entire body. Take time to yawn, stretch, and breathe deeply.

Remember to take off your shoes every hour during a long flight and exercise your ankles and toes.

When you arrive at your destination, give yourself a good half-hour workout of Hatha Yoga in your room so you can go into your day or evening refreshed and invigorated.

EXERCISES IN A WHEELCHAIR

People with severe disabilities can modify the postures. Even if you or a loved one is confined to bed, chances are they can do one or two things even if it's breathing and relaxation.

Start with simple shoulder and arm-and-neck movements. Then work up to the forward bends, etc., as you get stronger.

If possible, do the exercises with feet on the floor, not on your chair's foot supporter.

Caution: Remember to lock your brake before exercising so your chair does not move.

If you have a severe disability, start with simple breathing and relaxation before trying any of the movements.

Secure your doctor's approval before attempting any exercise.

"Everybody has a wheelchair: it is just that some people's wheelchairs are in their heads." (Larry Rossiter, quadriplegic; educational counselor, coordinator of Cincinnati College of Physical Medicine and Rehabilitation.)

THE 20-MINUTE ROUTINE FOR CHAIR-SITTERS

COMPLETE BREATH

Relax your jaw and be sure you have loosened the clothing around your neck, and close your mouth. Open your nostrils and back of the throat as if you were stifling a yawn.

Exhale all stale air out of lungs. Then inhale, slowly drawing air in through nose, not your mouth. Exhale, smoothly making exhalation longer than inhalation. This is one Complete Breath.

Repeat a few rounds of Complete Breath in between each exercise.

Read more about breathing in chapter 4.

MAKE A FACE

Placing tongue to roof of mouth close your eyes. Press the tongue to the roof of mouth. Hold a few seconds; relax the tongue.

Slide jaw gently from side to side.

Inhale. Hold the breath and purse your lips together; contract cheek muscles; squeeze eyebrows together. Exhale, releasing all tension from your face. Close eyes and observe the sensation within the face.

NECK PRESS

Place your right hand against your head above your right ear. Inhale. Then exhaling, press your head against your hand. Offer slight resistance with your hand. Release. Then bring your hand to your forehead and repeat the resistance. Release.

Repeat movement with left hand above left ear and then on the forehead. Exercise 2 times each direction.

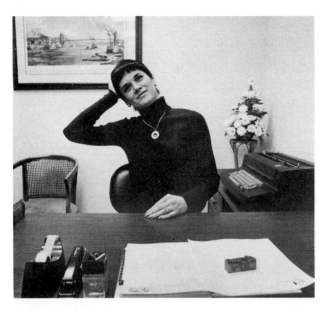

Neck Press

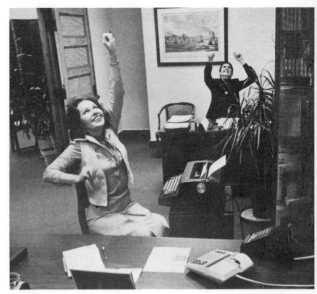

Picking Apples

ROW A BOAT

Raise arms directly in front of you, and make fists with hands as if to row a boat.

With elbows straight draw one shoulder back, then forward, and let the other arm follow as if rowing with straight arms. Repeat 5 to 10 times, while breathing comfortably.

As you come forward, push with the heel of the hand to get an extra stretch. Repeat 5 to 10 times.

STRETCH AND YAWN

Bring your arms above the head. (Perhaps, if you're in a plane or cramped quarters, bend elbows, cross wrists, resting hands behind neck.)

Slowly stretch one arm up toward ceiling; inhaling smoothly, open your mouth and yawn. Exhale and lower arm. This movement should feel good, so take your time. Repeat 3 or 4 times each side of body.

If arms are straight, push the ceiling away with the heels of hands.

OVER-THE-HEAD SPINE SCRATCH

Raise your right arm above head, bend your right elbow, and place right hand on spine as if to scratch between shoulders.

Bring your left hand up to right elbow and slowly and gently pull the bent elbow toward center of the head. Release. Repeat 3 times for each arm.

ARM CIRCLES

Arms in T position.

Make some large, slow circles in the air with fists clenched tightly.

Then make small circles in the air; be sure arms are as rigid as possible.

Bring arms across your chest and hug yourself. Inhale and open arms wide. Then exhaling, cross arms once again and give yourself a beautiful hug.

PICKING APPLES

Reach up as if to pick apples. Start at the lower braches; then work up to higher and higher branches. Inhale to reach up; release and stretch. Exhale.

SWIM

Bring arms above head and stretch and yawn. Then pretend to swim, extending arms in front of you.

BOUND STRETCH

Interlock hands in front of you; turn palms away from you and raise arms, palms facing ceiling as you stretch upward. Inhale and stretch up. Release, stretch, and exhale. Repeat on opposite side 2 or 3 times.

Lilias, Yoga, and Your Life

BACKSTROKE

Place fingertips on shoulders (right hand to right shoulder, left hand to left shoulder) with elbows together. Inhale, opening up elbows as wide as possible. Exhale, bringing elbows together. Repeat smoothly 3 to 6 times.

Using a swimmer's backstroke, make a large forward circle motion with elbows. Repeat 3 to 6 times.

HAND CIRCLES

With arms in front and elbows bent, make large, slow circles with hands. Take a few Complete Breaths. Relax shoulders. Repeat 5 times each direction.

HAND STARS

Open hands up like a large star. Hold the stretch and then release and make a fist. Repeat 5 times slowly. Observe sensation in hands.

PLAYING THE PIANO

Pretend to play the piano.
Make circles with your wrists.
Rub hands together vigorously.
Pretend you are washing hands. Now shake the water from your fingers.
Gently pull at individual fingers.

ELBOW-TO-KNEE POSE

Bend right elbow. Inhale. Then, exhaling, bring your left knee up to right elbow. Inhale and return to sitting position.
Repeat on opposite side.
Repeat 10 to 15 times.

SLALOM

Sit with heels as far right as possible. This is easy to do in a swivel-type chair. With knees together facing left, extend arms in front of you so you are right over your heels. Lift heels, swinging them briskly over to the left. Swing your arms in the same direction. Repeat 15 to 30 times.

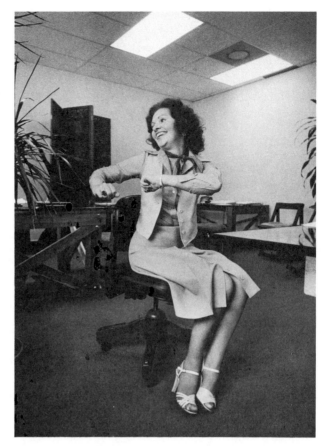

Slalom

HOLLOW LAKE

Sit with hands in lap. Look down at your hands. Inhale. Then exhale completely, holding the air out and drawing in your abdomen, toward your spine. Tighten your sphincter muscle. Hold five seconds. Release and repeat 3 to 5 times.

PELVIC TILT

Inhale. Then, exhaling, tighten your buttocks muscles and sphincter muscle, and pull stomach in firmly. Hold a few seconds. Release and relax all the muscles. Repeat 4 to 8 times.

THIGH AND BUTTOCKS FIRMER

Focus your attention on the thigh and buttocks muscle. Inhale, holding breath and contract thigh, buttocks and anal muscles. Hold 3 to 5 seconds. Release, breathe, and let muscles relax. Close your eyes; observe thighs. Repeat 3 to 5 times.

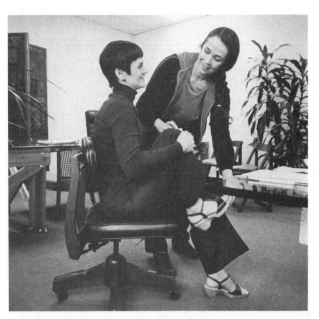
Seated Leg Lifts

SEATED LEG LIFTS

Take shoes off, if possible.

Tighten stomach muscles. Inhale. Bend your right knee and lift your right thigh off chair. Keep foot flexed throughout movement. Wrap arms around your knee and squeeze thigh to chest. Then straighten leg out in front of you. Hold onto arm rest for balance only. Use stomach muscles and lower thigh to chair. Repeat 3 times each leg.

FEET AND ANKLES

Cross thighs (not good for leg circulation to hold for long periods of time). Make a large circle with big toe by rotating ankle, 5 times each direction.

Repeat on opposite foot and ankle.

Pretend you are playing piano with your toes.

Jog in place while seated. Have a grand time. Move your arms. Pretend you are winning that marathon!

FOOT LIFT

Take off shoes if possible.

Bring both feet together.

Keeping the balls of feet on the floor, briskly lift your heels up and down 10 to 15 times.

Then lift just the toes and balls of feet off the floor. Then lift the heels. Briskly rock from heel to toe, 10 to 15 times.

ENTIRE BODY FIRMER

Place hands on armrests.

Keep knees bent.

Inhaling, tighten stomach muscle and push down on armrests and lift buttocks 2 inches off chair. Hold, breathing comfortably.

Release, relax and observe the feeling within entire body. Relax all muscles of the body.

Repeat.

SPINE CURL (FORWARD MOVEMENT)

Bring both arms above head; bend elbows; place hands behind neck, crossing wrists.

Inhale, stretching both elbows up to ceiling.

Exhale, bringing chin to throat.

Inhale and round your spine, shoulders, upper neck. Then exhale, and slowly lower your forehead to your knees. This entire movement should take 15 seconds.

Once your forehead is touching your knees, relax arms, hands to floor. Take a few deep breaths, relaxing muscles of lower back, shoulders, and abdomen.

Then slowly come up to a seated position. Repeat this spine curl 5 times.

PAT ON THE BACK

Sit tall, raise your left arm, reach *across* your chest, and give yourself a big pat on the back! Repeat 6 firm pats! Then repeat on the opposite shoulder.

SEATED CHEST EXPANDER

Sit at the edge of your chair.

Exhale, leaning way forward and bringing chest to thighs.

Clasp your hands behind you, thumbs comfortably touching lower back.

Straighten elbows, holding firmly onto hands.

Inhaling, sit slowly up, spine straight and wrists resting on chair back.

Exhale, lift chin up dropping head back to touch upper shoulders. Gently squeeze shoulder blades together. Hold position. Take one Complete Breath. Inhale; lift chest; exhale. Press shoulders together. Inhale deeply once again.

Then on exhalation, slowly bring chest to thigh once again. Release arms.

Sit up and close eyes and observe shoulders, arms,

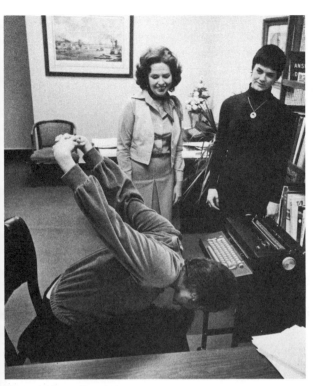

Seated Chest Expander

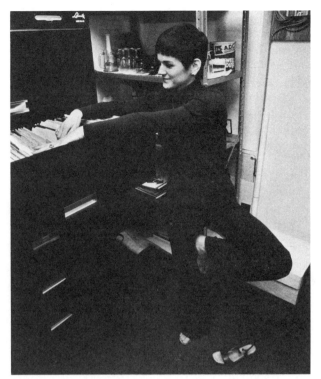

Tree at the Office

and neck. Visualize that all fatigue, stress, and strain are draining out of the fingertips.

This should feel good. However, if this feels uncomfortable or too strenous, don't force. Chest Expander *does* require some flexibility.

Repeat exercise 2 to 3 times.

TREE

Stand either at your desk or filing cabinets. Remove one shoe from your foot, reach down and grab that ankle and bring the heel of your foot either onto the inside of the opposite thigh or high on the inside of the same thigh. Stand tall, place your hand on the wall or cabinets for balance if needed. Rest the bent leg in this position for 15 to 30 seconds; then repeat on your opposite leg. Don't forget to put on your shoes! This is a very restful pose for those of you who stand on your legs all day and for those who do not move around.

SEATED SPONGE RELAXATION

Always end your exercise with relaxation. Close your eyes, rest hands in lap, and then consciously relax all parts of the body. If you can, take off shoes and start by relaxing toes and working up to each individual body part. First, focus your attention on that part of your body you wish to relax, such as the feet. Second, give continuous suggestions to the feet to relax. Third, feel the sensation of relaxation in those muscles you are relaxing.

After your feet are relaxed, go on to legs, then abdomen and pelvic region, spine, chest, arms, neck and then face. Spend at least a minute on each body part. It's also fun to be creative about your suggestion, such as, "I relax the bottom of my feet, and now I feel them melting into the floor."

It will help you tremendously to read chapters 3 and 12. Relaxation is a thought process and I think you will find it interesting, practical and usable for your everyday, busy life.

CIRCULATION PROBLEMS AND EXERCISE

Problems
Fatigue
Swelling of legs and ankles
Varicose veins
Cold hands and feet
Poor memory

Exercises
Hand Circles
Foot Circles

Shoulder Rolls
Slalom
Picking Apples
Row a Boat
Swim
Backstroke
Elbow-to-Knee Pose
Jogging in Place
Foot Lift

Over-the-Head Arm Clasp
Make a Face
Stretch and Yawn
Eye Rolls
Playing the Piano
Foot Circles

ABDOMINAL PROBLEMS AND EXERCISE

Problems
Digestion
Constipation
Prostate problems
Reduced muscle strength
Lower-back ache
Loss of abdominal tone

Exercises
Seated Sun Salutation 1 and 2
Thigh and Buttocks Firmer
Seat Tightener
Elbow-to-Knee Pose
Slalom
Hollow Lake
Pelvic Tilt
Knee to Chest
Spinal Twist
All forward bends
Stomach Lift

HAND, FACE, AND FEET PROBLEMS

Problems
Stiff shoulders
Stiff neck
Tired eyes
Lines in face and neck
Tension headaches
Neck and shoulder tension
Swollen ankles

Exercises
Neck Tilt
Shoulder Rolls
Lemon Squeeze

SPINE AND SHOULDER PROBLEMS

Problems
Dowager's hump
Lower-back ache
Shoulder tension
Stiff upper neck

Exercises
Lemon Squeeze
Spine Curl
Spinal Twist
Chest Expander
Shoulder Rolls
Triangle
Neck Tilt
Spine Curl
Hand Circles
Pat on the Back

TENSION THROUGHOUT BODY

Problems
Listlessness
Depression
Nervousness
Tension headache
Stiff neck
Burning sensation between shoulder blades

Exercises
Stretch and Yawn
Complete Breath
Shoulder Rolls
Triangle
Neck Press
Swim
Seated Chest Expander
Spine Curl
Row a Boat
Entire Body Firmer
Massage from Nice and Easy Yoga (Chapter 16)

Seated Sponge Relaxation
Read chapters 3 and 12

A Two-Minute Mini Office Yoga Break. Have Fun!

10:00 A.M.   Stretch and Yawn
           Spine Curl
           Neck Rolls
           Shoulder Rolls
           End all Yoga breaks with three Complete Breaths, seated in Relaxation. Breathe in energy. Breathe out fatigue.

11:00 A.M.   Picking Apples
           Pat on the Back
           Jog in place briskly. Smile.
           Stretch and Yawn
           Slalom

3:00 P.M.   3 Complete Breaths. Breathe in well-being. Breathe out the blahs.
           Shoulder Rolls

           Do 3 "All Shoulder Work" exercises
           Seated Chest Expander

4:00 P.M.   Jog in place briskly
           Neck Press
           Neck Tilt

5:00 P.M.   Seated Knee to Chest
Before   Entire Body Firmer
dinner   Spine Curl
           Tree
           3 Complete Breaths. Energy in. Tiredness out.
           Elbow-to-Knee Pose
           Backstroke

You should also read chapter 12, "Creative Stress—Creative Tension," and chapter 13, "Back Talk."

My thanks to Transport Systems, Inc., and their two affable secretaries, Joy Rolfsen and Mary Trippel, who have demonstrated these postures.

16
Nice and Easy Yoga

Yoga is for everyone, at any age. You can begin at any time of your life. If you are over 65 and an absolute beginner, welcome! There is no better time to start than this moment! You don't need to rush into a five-minute headstand or a difficult pose. Just start with the weekly practice schedule and do what makes you feel comfortable and good. Soon you will build up your confidence. Although most exercises are done on the floor, many can be done sitting in a chair or in your bed before you get up in the morning.

Hatha Yoga is great preventive medicine. When you start this program, you can expect to increase circulation to your head, arms, and legs. This may help normalize blood pressure and ease the strain on the heart.

The basic action within most Yoga postures is what is called squeeze, hold, release. For example, muscles, which surround the digestive organs, are asked to contract as you go into a Forward Bend. This contraction of muscles then massages or squeezes the digestive organs. You hold the position for a few seconds. Then you release it and a fresh supply of blood comes to the digestive and genital-urinary systems. Constipation problems therefore are allegedly helped with the deep, natural massage of the Yoga postures. With the increase of circulation comes an increase of health. In addition the breath-

ing exercises will increase the oxygen fed to all parts of the body, which will in turn raise your energy level.

Do these exercises any time during your day. You can do your Seated Leg Lifts while in the kitchen waiting for water to boil. Do your Foot Flaps while sitting on a bus. Try your relaxation and breathing while waiting in your dentist's office. Massage your shoulders while in the bathtub or pool. Take a stretch break in between hands of bridge. Do the Knee-to-Chest while you watch television.

If you are ill, you still can do quite a few simple exercises provided your doctor gives an okay. They will help you remain active and recuperate faster. If you have a cold, and breathing exercises and/or standing poses bother you, try the seated arm exercises or leg lifts, and Foot Flaps. If you are bedridden, there are Yoga exercises that can help relieve bedsores and constipation.

Yoga does not just help physically; it also teaches you to be positive in all conditions! Being positive feels good and uplifts your spirits as well as those of the people around you.

More doctors are becoming familiar with Yoga either through their enthusiastic patients or by personally taking classes.

I hope that in the years to come Hatha Yoga classes will be a part of all medical schools. Recently I received a warm and encouraging letter from a doctor in Chicago. He said, "Thank you, Lilias, for sharing these healthful exercises with so many. It makes my office waiting room less crowded." *To be on the safe side, be sure to check with your doctor before starting Yoga or any form of exercise.*

I also strongly recommend that you combine the exercise program with an improved diet, one that gives you the proper nutrition.

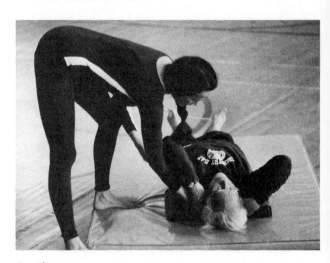

On Floor

To help you develop your higher self, and to quiet and unclutter your mind, I also suggest you try meditating (see page 126).

Many of my students, of all ages, have reported that meditation has become a welcome part of their daily routine; they have said that it adds richness and serenity to their lives.

A CASE HISTORY

Kathryn (Babe) Meier, 67, and Ed Meier, 71, parents of 5 children and grandparents of 10, have been in my classes for 3 years. They have shared their genuine enthusiasm and love of the Yoga exercises with all of us in the class.

Babe and Ed have enriched my life, and it gives me pleasure to introduce them to you. Kathryn Meier explains:

A few years ago I watched you on television. It was then I got started practicing Yoga. I had heard that Yoga exercises were good for arthritis, and I had severe arthritic problems. I had been in the hospital once for my hips and once for my knee, and I had very severe bursitis in each shoulder. So I thought maybe I would like to try those exercises.

Since I started practicing Yoga, I haven't been in the hospital, nor have I had a serious attack of bursitis.

I also want to tell you how much Yoga has helped my nerves. I used to get nervous about little and big things. When I was in the hospital with pancreatitis a while back, no one thought I'd live through the night. As the doctors and nurses rushed around, I realized I could worry or I could relax. I chose to relax, and I think it pulled me through.

My friends noticed that I'm thinner. I must be 15 pounds lighter than I was before Yoga, and I'm down three dress sizes. My Yoga gives me the incentive to watch my diet and do my exercises each day.

At the end of my routine and relaxation, I feel as if I'm just floating. You know, I could love Yoga just because of that.

Ed Meier says it was his wife who persuaded him to attend the Yoga class.

I had problems with my shoulder and the back of my neck. The tension in my neck really was very bad. I used to rub ointment on my neck every night. In my job I'd drive a long way and travel a whole lot. It tensed me up. Now I think Yoga has taken care of most of that!

I also had arthritis so bad in this shoulder that my arm felt frozen. It was awful! I couldn't get my hands up high enough to put a token in the toll box going across the bridge. After a year of my Yoga exercises, I can go up to here!

Oh yes, it keeps me young and thinking clearer. I'm less tired. We do a lot of walking together, but that's not enough.

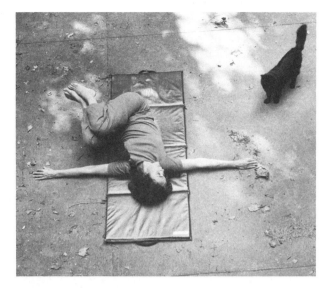
Lilias Enjoying a Posture

I see lots of improvement in Babe. She's more ambitious around the house. She really wants to get out and *do* things. Always wants to be in the yard. In the morning she can't wait to see the daylight so she can get out and get going!

Helpful Hints

The best time of day to practice your Yoga routine is whenever it's best for you!

Some men and women like to start their day with Yoga. It gives them pep and optimism. Others enjoy closing the day with Yoga to release any tensions or fatigue.

Set aside a time for practice; then *stick to it*! It is better to do 10 or 15 minutes each day, than to miss four days and try to catch up with longer sessions.

If you do miss a few days, don't get discouraged; just keep on going!

Stop while you're having fun and everything feels good to you. Don't *ever* push yourself to pain.

Dress comfortably.

Find a quiet place to exercise and close the door and take the phone off the hook so you won't be disturbed. Pets too can be a distraction, so it's best to remove them from the room. For excessive stiffness, try taking a warm bath before and after exercising; also try massaging your own stiff knees, shoulders, and feet. For excessive stiffness in the hip, try sitting on a pillow while in the Forward Bend (for details see page 61). For excessive stiffness in the back of the leg, try doing Leg Raises with a Necktie, or bend your knees in Forward Bend. For excessive stiffness in the spine, or for discomfort during relaxation, try placing a pillow beneath your knees, a rolled-up hand towel in the curve of your upper neck, and/or a small pillow beneath your head.

Nice and Easy Yoga

DAILY REMINDER

Tape the following list to your bathroom mirror and on the refrigerator door as a reminder. Each day I am going to do the following:

I will bend, stretch, and rotate my legs, arms, spine, chest, and abdomen.

I will gently twist my spine and neck area side to side, forward, and backward.

I will massage my internal organs and glands by doing a daily Forward Bend and a Stomach Lift.

I will invert myself daily in a way that is right for my body.

I will take time each day to breathe deeply and relax my body, to calm my mind and my emotions.

Slowly and surely I will gain in my confidence and poise.

I will make this day a better day for someone else.

WEEKLY PRACTICE SCHEDULE

This is a simple practice schedule for the man or woman, over 65, who has not exercised for many years. But understand that there are students who are over 65 in regular classes, doing the *same* program with other students who are 30 years younger. This is a goal you might like to set for yourself.

Meanwhile, start with the first week. Stay with the first week until you are comfortable and confident. Let one exercise flow smoothly into the other. with breathing in between. Start seated in a chair if you'd like; then move onto your non-skid exercise mat. Repeat the first week as a warmup each time, as you go to the second week, then the third, etc. Always remember to end with breathing and a 5-minute Relaxation.

Week One

All the following exerises are warmups:
Neck Roll
Shoulder Roll
Single Shoulder Roll
Hand Circles
Make a Face
Massage your body
Face Tap and Ear Pulls
3 Complete Breaths seated

Hand Circles
Eye Exercises
Seated Leg Lifts
Foot Circles
Foot Flaps
Arm Circles
Stretch and Yawn
Lemon Squeeze
Side Stretch
Seated Knee-to-Chest Squeeze
3 Complete Breaths, lying down
Easy Seated Twist
Seated Sun Salutation 1 & 2
Complete Breath
Humming Breath and Meditation
3 Complete Breaths in Sponge
Seated Sponge Relaxation

Week Two

All warmups from Week One
Bump
Forehead to Knee
Seated Triangle
Easy Twist
Leg Lifts
Humming Breath and Meditation
Seated Sponge Relaxation
Read Chapter 3 on Relaxation. Relax 5 minutes.

Week Three

All warmups from Week One
Relax in Sponge—take 6 Complete Breaths.
Add the following new exercises:
Locust 1 and 2
Phoenix 1 and 2
Pose of a Child
Humming Breath and Meditation
Seated Sponge Relaxation—5 minutes
Read Chapter 13, "Back Talk"

Week Four

All warmups from Week One
Rock-and-Roll
Easy Bridge
Abdominal Lift
Humming Breath and Meditation
Seated Sponge Relaxation—5 minutes

Week Five

All warmups from Week One
All Standing Poses
Forward Bend
Humming Breath and Meditation
Breathing
Seated Sponge Relaxation—5 minutes

Week Six

All warmups from Week One
Half Candle
Easy Fish
Humming Breath and Meditation
Breathing
Seated Sponge Relaxation—5 minutes

First Week

NECK ROLL

Start by sitting slightly forward in a chair, with knees apart, arms very relaxed, hanging straight down toward the floor. Rest your hands comfortably on knees and hold your head straight in center position.

Exhale and lower chin to the throat.

Inhale and gently lift chin and drop head back. Very slowly repeat this forward-backward movement 3 times.

Bring head back to center.

Exhale, lowering right ear to right shoulder. Inhale and go to center. Exhale, lower left ear to left shoulder. Inhale, bring head back to center. Repeat 3 times.

Make a complete circle with head, starting with chin to throat. Then rotate to right shoulder, back, and left shoulder, in slow, smooth, continuous movement. When done, close eyes and note sensation in neck area.

Roll 3 times in each direction.

SHOULDER ROLL

Inhaling, bring shoulders slowly toward ears. Exhale, lower shoulders slowly back to normal position. Repeat 3 times.

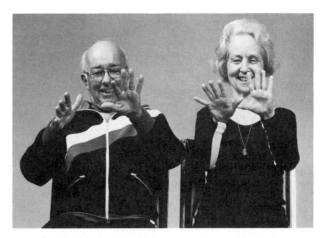

Play the Piano with Your Fingers

Now move shoulders in a circle by rotating them back, then up under the ears, and then forward and down to normal position.

Proceed with Shoulder Roll 3 times in each direction.

Repeat the rolls on opposite shoulder.

SINGLE SHOULDER ROLL

Sit straight and lift right shoulder up under right ear. Then roll your shoulder in a circle, back, down, forward and up. Repeat the circle with right shoulder in the opposite direction. Then repeat with left shoulder in each direction.

MAKE A FACE

Close eyes; observe how face muscles feel. Inhale and gently pursing mouth together, squeeze eyes closed and squeeze eyebrows together. Hold a comfortable 3 to 5 seconds. Release and observe the difference in how your face feels. Repeat.

FACE TAPS AND EAR PULLS

Exhale, release, relax, and observe the warmth, tingle in muscles and skin of face.

For a few seconds gently tap forehead with fingers; then tap cheeks, and massage your temples. Don't rush.

Grasp ear lobes, pulling them down and then releasing them. Repeat 6 times. Then grasp top of ears and lift them. Release. Repeat 6 times.

With middle finger, lightly touch the inside of ear as if you were feeling the inside of a shell. Be curious. Spend a few seconds doing this. Then massage firmly the hard bone behind the back of ear.

Rest hands in lap. Close the eyes. Observe face and ears.

MASSAGE

Massaging your joints and muscles each day helps remove the aches and pains from stiffness and helps increase your circulation. First briskly rub hands together, creating warmth and energy. Then start with face and ears. Work down to rubbing shoulders, head, neck, elbows, lower back, knees, hands, and feet. Rub in a firm, circular motion. Use the full length of the fingers, creating warmth. Then massage the area of skin around the joints. This is easy to do while watching television.

EYE EXERCISES

Sit comfortably in your chair. Remove glasses, if you are wearing them, and look straight ahead.

Open eyes wide, but do not strain.

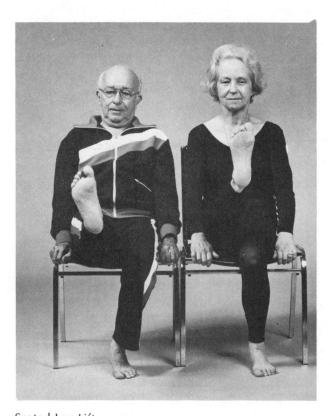

Seated Leg Lifts

Look up to ceiling through eyebrows, but don't move your head.

Look down over your cheekbones to your lap.

Bring eyes back to center position.

Look to the right, as if you were trying to see over your right shoulder without moving your head. Bring eyes to center. Then, look over the left shoulder without moving your head.

Repeat entire process 3 times.

Next roll the eyes in slow, large circles, first to the right, then down to floor, then to left, then up to ceiling. Repeat the circular movement in opposite direction. Then close eyes.

Rub palms together to warm them.

Then, press flat palms gently over the eyeballs. Release; then press again. This gentle pressure helps relax the eye muscles when they are tired.

Next, hold arm directly in front of face with index finger raised. Focus on your finger; then slowly focus on a spot across the room. Return focus to the fingertip again; then return focus to wall. Go back and forth several times; then close eyes and then rest them. Observe the sensation in and around the eyes. Breathe slowly in and out.

Helpful Hints
Do not turn or move head.
Do not overstrain eyes.

SEATED LEG LIFTS

Grasp the chair seat with hand. Inhale and raise the right leg up, knee as straight as possible. Hold 3 seconds. Exhaling, lower the right foot to floor. Repeat process 3 to 8 times for each leg.

FOOT CIRCLES

Grasping the chair seat with both hands, raise the right leg up. Then make a circle with the foot and ankle. Try to draw a zero with your big toe.

Repeat on opposite leg. Work up to 3 each side.

FOOT FLAPS

Sit and hold on to the edge of the chair, or sit on a mat with legs straight out. Flex your feet by extending your heel. Observe how the skin stretches on the bottom of the feet; then straighten the foot by arching the foot and gently pointing your toe. Repeat this motion 10 to 15 times with one foot at a time; then both feet.

Be careful about squeezing your toes too vigorously. This often causes foot cramps. If you do get a foot cramp or charley horse, then firmly press your finger beneath your nose, above your lip. We don't know why it works, but it seems to help this problem.

Raise arms to shoulder level in T position.

Make 3 to 5 large, slow circles with arms rigid; then reverse the directions. Be sure arms are rigid. Then make smaller, faster circles. Reverse the direction.

SIDE STRETCH

Inhale and raise arms toward ceiling. Exhale, slowly and gently bend to the right. Inhale and return to center. Exhale and bend gently to the left. Repeat bend on each side.

Lower arms and close eyes. Take a slow breath in and out. Observe.

SEATED KNEE-TO-CHEST SQUEEZE

Inhale deeply and bring bent right knee to chest by grasping arms around your lower leg.

Exhale and squeeze thigh to chest and abdomen. Bring nose close to knee. Hold for 3 to 5 seconds. Breathing comfortably lower leg to floor, exhaling.

Take a smooth breath in and out; then repeat on opposite leg. Repeat 5 times each side.

EASY SEATED TWIST

Sit comfortably in straight-backed chair, sitting slightly forward, not leaning against the chair back.

Knees are together and straight out in front of you. Place right hand on your left knee. Place left hand over the chair back.

Inhale; then, exhaling, gently twist to the left. Start from the navel to the left, then ribs, then left shoulder, then chin, then eyes, looking way over left shoulder. Hold position 10 seconds, breathing comfortably.

Then slowly return to center position, feeling each part of the body as it returns forward.

Repeat procedure 2 to 3 times in each direction.

Helpful Hints

Keep eyes open and feet on the floor.

Twist gently and slowly. This is not a quick movement.

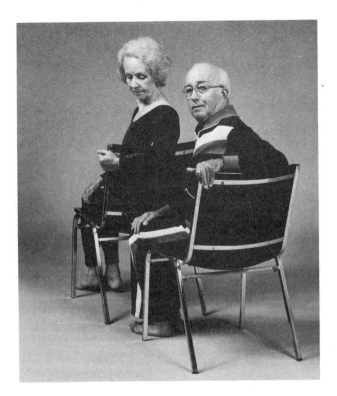

Easy Seated Twist

SEATED SUN SALUTATION 1

Sitting straight bring knees together.

Exhale, bend forward, laying chest on thighs.

Clasp hands to elbows. Bring arms around knees.

Hold position, breathing comfortably for 3 to 5 seconds.

Inhale and come up to straight position, still holding elbows.

Exhale and lower arms. Repeat 3 times.

After you get used to this Seated Sun Salutation, learn to hold this pose up to 30 seconds. You will find it relaxing for lower back.

SEATED SUN SALUTATION 2

Sit forward, away from chair's back. Spread knees as far apart as comfortable.

Inhale slowly through nose and raise your arms over head. Exhale and slowly bend forward, between knees, toward the floor.

Go as far as you can toward the floor without strain. Soon both hands will touch the floor.

Hold comfortably in position, relaxing face and neck.

Then inhale, slowly raising the arms above head.

Exhale and lower hands to lap. Close eyes. Observe sensation within body.

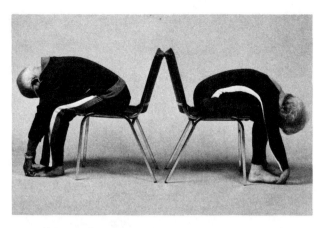

Seated Sun Salutation

Repeat procedure 3 to 5 times.

Helpful Hints

Breathe in and out through nose.

Breathe and move body together.

Try the Bhrumeri Breath with this pose. (See page 13 and below on this page.) Hum as you go forward.

COMPLETE BREATH

Complete Breath (see chapter 4, page 13) can be done anywhere—in your car at stoplights, while waiting for lunch at a restaurant, sitting at the edge of a pool, lying in bed before sleep.

It is called Complete Breath because you are required to use both the upper and lower parts of your lungs. It is this unique combination that helps you receive the most out of your total lung capacity.

Let a few cycles of Complete Breath separate each exercise.

Helpful Hints

Do *not* slouch to exhale. This is cheating your muscles out of the work they so desperately need to stay healthy.

Practice this exercise daily, perhaps five cycles in the morning and five in the evening. Very soon you will really enjoy it!

Observe within yourself the positive results of this wonderful breath in your life. Feel how it rejuvenates and soothes the entire nervous system.

Imagine breathing in light, health, energy, strength, healing, and clarity of mind, and imagine exhaling all negativity, heaviness, toxins, and tensions of body, mind, and spirit.

Realize that this exercise is possibly the *most important* item of your daily practice; you are feeding your body, mind, and spirit.

HUMMING BREATH AND MEDITATION

I have always enjoyed how Humming Breath makes me feel. I like the sound vibration as it flows through my mouth, neck, and chest. I also like how it relaxes me. I'm sure you'll enjoy it too!

Humming Breath helps your mind to focus on the breathing process and slows down the stiff exhalation by giving you something to push against. You simply inhale smoothly, mouth closed, relaxing your jaw and tongue, opening the back of the throat (as if stifling a yawn). After filling your lungs completely, exhale by singing out the breath with a *hum* sound. The *hum* sound should have as prolonged an *m* as possible. It sounds like the gentle *hum-m-m* of a bee. Try to keep one continuous tone from beginning to end as you exhale totally *all* air from lungs.

Then inhale once again smoothly and quietly, and on the exhalation repeat the Humming Breath. The eyes are closed. The face is relaxed. After you have done Humming Breath for a few minutes, relax your hands in your lap. Imagine that you are emptying your body and mind of all tensions, negatives and worries. Suggest to your entire body that it relaxes from this sitting position. Remain calm and alert; resist the temptation to doze. Observe the mind and watch your thoughts as they flow in and out of your head. Soon they will quiet down.

As you sit quietly, and experience the inner peacefulness of your mind and body, feel the peace with each effortless breath that flows in and out of your lungs. Sink deeper into its warmth, into its light, into its calmness. Feel it expand in your chest, throat, and head. *Feel* it surround you and envelop you. Remain still and calm within the experience for a comfortable 5 to 20 minutes.

Observe the surface of your mind, as if you were looking at a smooth, quiet lake; move this surface of your mind with a positive thought with each breath—health, joy, love, and inner balance; on your exhalation imagine sending these thoughts to every cell of your body. The breath is acting like a messenger, taking this positive energy to all the cells that need nourishment and healing. This is a very simple but effective meditation that will tune and sharpen the mind and spirit. This is also a lovely way to conclude your time of prayer.

Helpful Hints

Take the phone off hook and remove pets from room during meditation time.

Let your family know you do not wish to be disturbed for a few minutes.

Do *not* strain or force this technique.

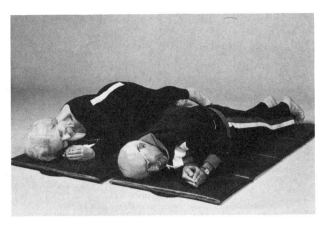

Bump

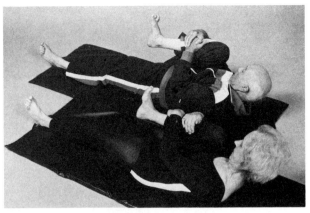

Forehead to Knee—Lying on the Mat

Let your impatience go.

Do not look for instant results.

Trust that all is in perfect attunement and harmony.

Because complete relaxation is very important, I suggest you read pages 10–11 on the three steps to relaxation. In fact read it over many times until it becomes a part of you. Also review the meditation techniques here and on pages 84–85.

The Seated Sponge Relaxation pose (page 117) can be one of the strongest aids I know of in a time of upheaval as well as in a time of serenity.

Second Week

This is not a traditional Yoga exercise. It is designed to help you move around on the floor with confidence and also to limber up your body. Have some fun with it!

BUMP

Lie on right side, arms and hands in front of chest; then roll onto your stomach, hands in front of your chest. Tucking your left shoulder completely under you, roll over to left side.

Go back and forth several times, letting your arms pull you through.

FOREHEAD TO KNEE LYING ON THE MAT

Step 1
Lie on back with arms alongside body.

Bend right knee to chest. Clasp hands over lower leg. Holding below the knee and breathing comfortably, press the knee to chest and hold for 10 sec-

onds before releasing. Relax your shoulders and face. Hold pose but *not* the breath.

Still holding the knee to chest, gently pull the bent leg out to the side, over rib cage. Release leg and return it to the starting position.

Repeat on opposite side.

Step 2
Exhaling, clasp knee to chest and raise the forehead up toward the knee. Hold 3 to 5 seconds. Breathing comfortably, release and relax.

Repeat 3 times each side. Observe. Remind yourself to relax shoulders.

As you become more proficient, try both knees to chest.

Helpful Hints
Do not hold breath during this exercise.

Pause before you go to other leg and feel the difference in one leg as compared to the other.

SEATED TRIANGLE

Sit in your chair, hips facing forward. Raise arms to a T position. Inhale; then as you exhale bring the left hand down to your right foot. Raise right hand up to the ceiling. Look up to the thumb on your right hand and hold 3 to 5 seconds, breathing comfortably.

Inhale and come back up to T.

Exhale and repeat with opposite arm.

Repeat the entire procedure once more.

EASY TWIST

Sit tall on your mat with legs straight out in front of you. Place left hand over the right knee.

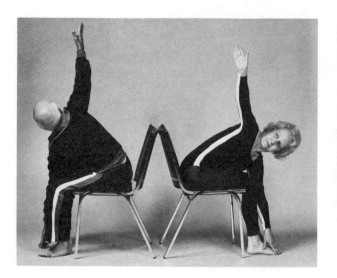

Seated Triangle

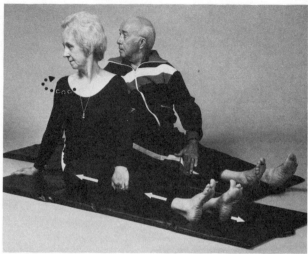

Easy Twist

Raise the right arm up to the ceiling; then place the fingertips of the right hand behind you on the mat. Thumb toward the spine.

Start the Easy Twist by extending the left heel slightly forward and allowing right heel to move back.

Inhale and sit tall. Then, exhaling, twist slowly to the right. Feel the navel first move to right, followed by ribs, then right shoulder, then chin, nose, and eyes.

Hold this pose, breathing comfortably, and apply gentle pressure to right knee with hand for 10 to 15 seconds. Then, slowly release each part of the body, starting with eyes, nose, etc.

Repeat the twist to left. Repeat exercise 1 to 2 times each direction.

LEG LIFTS

Lying on mat; bend both knees, feet flat to floor.

Inhale deeply; then, exhaling, tighten buttocks and gently press the arch from lower back. Keeping left foot flat to floor and left knee bent smoothly raise your right leg up toward ceiling with foot flexed.

Inhale again, then exhaling, lower right leg to floor.

Repeat 3 times on each leg. Work up to 6 each side.

Helpful Hints

Tighten seat muscles to protect lower back in leg raises.

Keep opposite foot on floor for leg raises, especially if lower back is weak.

Move slowly. Try Humming Breath as you lower leg. It will help you to slow down movement.

Third Week

LOCUST 1

Caution: This is not an exercise to do if you have a history of serious back problems.

Roll a towel into a firm roll, or use a small, hard pillow. Place it slightly below the hipbone.

Lie prone on your mat. Bring feet together. Place forehead on floor.

Place arms alongside your body, hands flat to floor.

Take one Complete Breath.

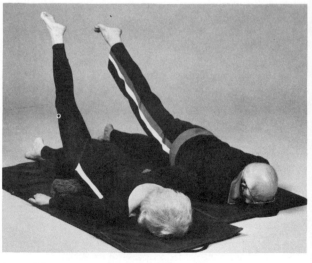

Locust I

Lilias, Yoga, and Your Life

Exhale, tilt the pelvis and raise right leg as high as possible.

Hold 3 to 5 seconds. Exhale and lower leg to floor.

Repeat 3 times each leg. After a few weeks, try lifting both legs together.

LOCUST 2

Move towel slightly above hipbone.

Exhale, lift head, arms, and chest. Legs rest on the floor. Continue raising arms and chest as high as possible while exhaling. Tighten buttocks firmly, and tilt the pelvis.

Inhale and smoothly lower arms to floor. *Do not* strain.

Helpful Hints

Avoid jerky movements. Lift and lower slowly. Eyes are open; gaze is steady.

Variation

Do remove towel and try lifting arm and leg together.

PHOENIX 1

Lying on the abdomen, bend elbows and place wrists beneath shoulders, fingertips facing forward, palms down. Keep upper arms close to body.

Tuck chin to throat and try to look for navel. Then slowly raise forehead, nose, and chin. Raise head up and back as far as possible. Tighten seat muscles and tilt the pelvis; press gently down on elbows and wrists, and lift chest even higher. Breathe comfortably and keeping lower arms on floor. (This is called the top of the pose.)

Slowly lower the head toward hands, tucking in the chin toward throat. Repeat 3 times.

PHOENIX 2

Repeat entire pose as directed above. This time hold at top of this pose, breathing comfortably. Hold between 10 to 30 seconds. Then lower the head between the hands.

Raise the head up once again.

Breathing comfortably, slowly turn your head and look over your right shoulder. Hold a few seconds; then look over the left shoulder.

Repeat and slowly lower forehead to floor.

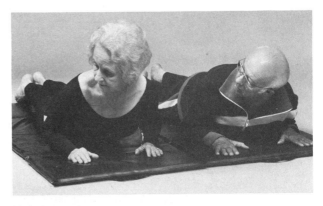

Phoenix 2

Helpful Hints

Move slowly; take 5 to 10 seconds to get to top of pose.

Breathe gently and use breath to lift you up.

Use hands as gentle leverage.

Tighten buttocks muscles as you arch your back.

POSE OF A CHILD

On a mat or in bed, fold legs beneath you by bending knees; bring knees together and sit on heels.

Inhale; then exhale slowly and bend forward lowering stomach to thighs. Place arms alongside your body, wrists close to ankles.

Relax deeply. Breathe comfortably.

Feel the tension and tightness leaving your shoulders, lower back, and upper neck.

Hold for as long as is comfortable.

Sit up without using arms.

Helpful Hints

Some people find it very uncomfortable to sit on their ankles. If so, simply place a pillow over ankles and heels; then sit on the pillow. This is a very comfortable resting pose, so please don't skip over it.

Variation

Place knees wide apart, with big toes touching before beginning the pose. This variation is extremely soothing for lower back.

Fourth Week

ROCK-AND-ROLL

Lying on a mat or bed, bring both knees to chest and wrap the arms behind the knees. Hold on firmly to one of your wrists.

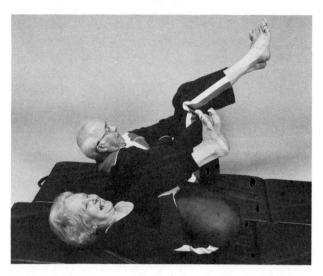

Rock and Roll

Inhale, then exhale and come up into a sitting position. At first, everyone feels a little stuck and awkward trying to sit up. Try lifting hips off the mat just a quarter inch, and start the rocking motion from there. Spend time getting in touch with this lying, rocking position. Feel the massage it is giving your lower back. Then, when you are more confident, bring your heels downward vigorously toward the back of your thighs. This kick should give you the momentum to sit up all the way, and rock and roll 3 times. Work up to 10.

EASY BRIDGE

Lying on your back, bend your knees, keeping them 12 inches apart (not beyond your hips), toes facing forward.

Press arch of spine to floor. Slowly, *one vertebra at a time*, raise the lower back to the middle of shoulders. Inhale as you go up.

Exhaling slowly, lower spine down to mat, *one vertebra at a time*.

Repeat 3 times.

Helpful Hints

Move slowly; breathe deeply and smoothly through nose.

Keep shoulders on mat.

Completely relax neck and throat throughout exercise.

ABDOMINAL LIFT

Go onto all fours. Let abdomen relax toward

floor and concave lower spine. Inhale fully so lungs expand.

Now exhale by opening the mouth, exhaling briskly, removing and emptying all the air from lungs. Hold breath out. Close the mouth and bring chin to throat gently.

Do not breathe in immediately. Pull your stomach in and out with a quick motion 5 to 6 times. Get in touch with this in-and-out motion of the abdominal muscle. Once you feel comfortable, and it comes easily, proceed further.

Go through the above steps, but this time, push down on heels of hands and arch spine like a cat.

As you do this motion, suck in abdomen as far as possible toward your spine. I call this a mock inhalation because you pretend to breathe in, but do not.

Hold 2 to 4 seconds. Then relax the abdomen toward the floor, inhaling deeply.

Repeat 3 to 6 times. Add on more as your strength and flexibility increase.

Helpful Hints

Exhale *completely* before you pull abdomen up and in. Resist the temptation to breathe.

Do not do this exercise after eating a meal.

CAUTION: *Do not* do this exercise after recent abdominal surgery or if there is a history of even mild heart disease.

Fifth Week

STANDING POSES (SIMPLE BALANCE WARMUP)

Standing behind a chair, lean forward, and place hands lightly on chair's back for support.

Inhale and lift the right leg to the back. Hold 3 seconds.

Exhale and release leg back to floor.

Repeat 3 to 6 times each leg.

Helpful Hints

Do not make this a jerky motion.

Variation

Do try this one in a swimming pool.

SIMPLE BALANCE POSE

Repeat above procedure and balance.

Keep eyes focused on an immovable spot six feet in front of you.

Hold pose 5 to 10 seconds, breathing comfortably.

Release and bring foot to floor gently.

Repeat with opposite leg.

STANDING LEG LIFTS

With right side facing a chair, place right hand on back of chair. Stand straight and tall.

Inhale and lift the leg up in front of you as high as possible without bending at the waist. Hold 3 seconds. Exhale and lower leg to floor. Repeat leg lift 3 times.

Inhale and raise leg out to side. Hold 3 seconds. Lower and repeat to side 3 times.

Raise leg to the back, hold, and repeat lift 3 times.

Raise leg to the front, hold and repeat lift 3 times.

Turn and, with the left side facing the chair, repeat Leg Lift with opposite leg in all directions, three times each direction.

Build up to 6 lifts each side.

This is an excellent exercise to do in the swimming pool.

TREE

With your left hand, hold onto a chair, wall, kitchen counter, or side of a pool.

Reach down and clasp your right ankle and draw right foot up and place the sole of the foot on the *inside* of left thigh or knee.

Raise the right arm overhead. Steady your balance by breathing shallowly and gazing at a spot on the floor about 6 feet in front of you.

Slowly raise left hand off chair a few inches. Hold there and breathe gently.

Once you have your balance, raise both arms above the head.

Come down slowly and in control.

Repeat the same process on other leg.

Helpful Hints

Move slowly from one movement to the other.

Keep focus on an immovable spot in front of you.

I suggest that after you have finished your standing poses, you try a simple Forward Bend. It is not a difficult posture and is exceedingly healthful. It gives a deep massage to all the abdominal organs as well as good stretch to the backs of the legs and lower back.

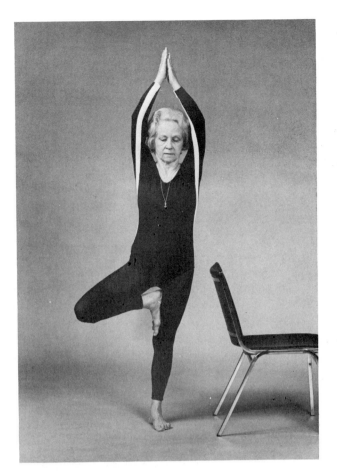

Tree Pose

Sixth Week—Inverted Pose

HALF CANDLE (HALF SHOULDERSTAND)

Please do not rush into the Half Candle (also known as the Half Shoulderstand). I cannot emphasize this enough!

To do the Half Candle needs some specific warm-ups. Rock and Roll is terrific to quickly warm and stretch out the muscles of the upper back, shoulders, and neck. Another good warmup is the Head Lift. Start with one rotation of the head side to side; then work slowly up to two each side.

Step 1

Place the front of the non-skid mat close to the wall. Sit sideways, hip about 3 to 4 inches from the wall; lean back and come to elbows.

Step 2

Turn so you face the wall, and raise the legs, resting the heels on the wall. Then lie down comfortably resting heels on the wall, buttock close to the wall, arms alongside the body.

Rest in this position for a few minutes. Feel the blood come gently to the chest and face, nourishing the skin, eyes, and brain.

Step 3

Press the soles of feet into the wall.

Raise buttocks off the mat by pushing slowly with feet into the wall and straightening legs.

Bend elbows and slide hands up to hips firmly. (Note Babe's hand position.)

Step 4

Raise one foot off wall and over head; opposite foot is still on wall. (Note Babe's foot position.)

Keeping elbows together as close as possible start to feel your balance in this position.

Step 5

Gently draw the other foot away from the wall bringing both feet together above your head. Your hands support your hips with ease. Neck and shoulders are comfortable and free of any pain. Your breathing is comfortable.

Hold pose for 10 to 20 seconds. As you get used to this inverted pose, you will enjoy holding the position longer.

To come out of the pose, simply lower one foot to wall, then the other foot. Please do not lower both legs at same time.

Variation

Follow this inverted pose with the Easy Fish Pose. The Fish will relieve lower-back tightness, and open, stretch, and stimulate the thyroid area around the throat.

EASY FISH POSE

As you become more confident in this inverted pose and the body becomes stronger (this may take weeks or months; just don't rush through the different stages—enjoy them!), move away from the wall and roll up into the Half Candle. To come down, place arms on the mat and use hands as brakes. Keep the knees close to chest, back of the head to the mat, and roll down slowly.

If you feel a slight pull in the lower back when resting, after this pose, lie on the mat, bring your knees to your chest and clasp knees. The pull is normal, and this discomfort goes away as your back gets stronger.

POSE OF TRANQUILITY

After you have worked up to holding the Half Candle, without using the wall then try this variation.

Go into Half Candle confidently.

Remove elbows from the mat and place hands on your thighs or knees and balance on your shoulders.

Breathe comfortably as you hold your shoulder-point-of-balance.

Come out of this pose by following the same procedure as in Half Candle.

Lie down and relax.

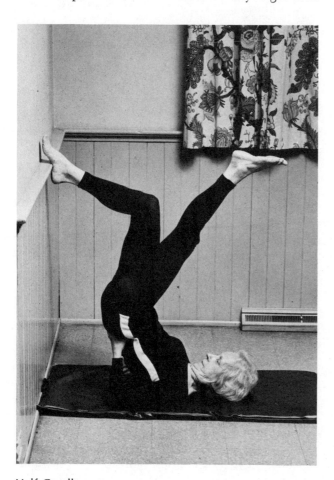

Half Candle

POISE, BALANCE, AND COORDINATION

Problems
Poor balance
Weak hips
Poor coordination and confidence

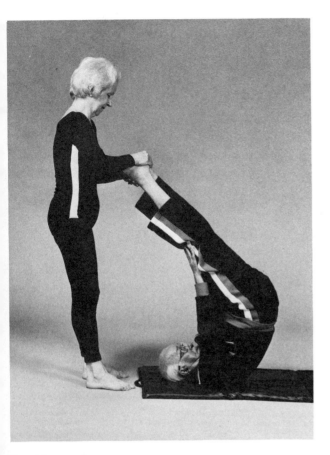

Shoulderstand

Exercises
Bump
All leg lifts
All standing poses
All inverted poses

NECK, FACE, AND EYES

Problems
Stiff neck
Tired eyes
Lines in face and neck
Weak and sagging neck muscles
Tension headaches
Neck and shoulder tension

Exercises
Stretch and Yawn
Neck Rolls
Eye exercises
Phoenix

All twists
Pose of a Child
Half Candle
Lemon Squeeze
Massage your body
Ear Pulls
Inverted Poses
Forward Bend

OVERWEIGHT AND POOR MUSCLE TONE

Problems
Paunchy stomach
Heavy hips
Flabby upper arms
Double chin
Thick ankles

Exercises
Neck Roll
Arm Circles
Leg Raise
Foot Circles
Knee-to-Chest Squeeze
Forward Bend
Easy Twist
Abdominal Lift
Locust 1 and 2

BACK, SHOULDERS, AND LEGS

Problems
Dowager's hump
Lower-back ache
Tension in shoulders
Sagging buttocks
Stiffness in legs
Stiffness in joints
Arthritic joints
Bursitis
Sciatica
Low stamina
Curvature of spine

Exercises
Massage the Body
Read chapters 3 and 12

Read chapter 13, "Back Talk"
Lemon Squeeze
Seated Forward Bend
Seated Triangle
Seated Sun Salutation 1 and 2
Foot Flaps
Locust 1 and 2
Shoulder Roll and Shrug
Easy Bridge
Rock-and-Roll
Phoenix 1 and 2

Pose of a Child
Rag Doll
Rolling Over and Back Up
Half Candle
All back exercises from chapter 13

Note. The preceding list is not meant to be an instant cure-all or a replacement treatment for your medical therapy. It is merely a summary of the exercises that teachers and students have found helpful in complementing control of certain problems.

To you dear friend, who asks the question, "Is it safe for me to study Hatha Yoga now that I am pregnant?" let me say how wonderful it is that you are about to embark upon this new phase of your journey. After you have asked your doctor if you can start or continue Yoga, and the answer is yes, then let us proceed together.

Yoga is not necessary during pregnancy, but it does help in many ways. If you are a seasoned Hatha student who feels like continuing with your usual practice, simply modify some Asanas slightly in order to continue reaping the benefits of Yoga. If you are just starting the Asanas during pregnancy, you have much to look forward to. Realize, though, that your study will not guarantee a perfect, problem-free delivery. What you can count on is sleeping better, keeping body tone, releasing negative tensions, gaining confidence during the delivery, and heightening self-knowledge.

If you are a beginner, I suggest you start with two or three stretches each morning and evening that make you feel happy and alive. I hope these two or three will lead to more, always followed by a breathing and relaxation time.

In addition to giving prenatal stretches, I have included a schedule for post-partum Yoga, which I hope you will also find helpful.

Interview with a Physical Therapist

Judith H. Lasater is a registered physical therapist with a Ph.D. from the California Institute of Asian Studies in San Francisco. In addition to contributing regularly to the *Yoga Journal*, she teaches at the Institute for Yoga Teacher Education, conducts workshops throughout the country, and is a Bradley natural-childbirth instructor.

Lilias: How many years had you studied Yoga before you became pregnant?

Judith: I started six and one-half years before.

Lilias: And then you continued with your study?

Judith: Yes I did. I did only as much as I felt like doing, such as with the Forward Bends, until the baby got in the way. I gave up back bends at 4 months because I felt too much tugging at the breastbone from overstretching the abdominal muscles.

Lilias: What did you learn from your training in natural birth?

Judith: One thing I had learned from my training was that as soon as one becomes pregnant, there is a large hormonal response, when a hormone called relaxin is produced by the pituitary gland. When pregnancy occurs, relaxin is released and has an effect on the whole body system. It causes the smooth muscles to relax and this has ramifications. It causes joints and ligaments to be looser. It causes you to lose some of the abdominal muscle tone. For example, the muscles of your digestive system, those muscles that help move food along, are more relaxed during pregnancy. One of the reasons for digestive problems during pregnancy is that the muscles at the top of your stomach aren't really tight. Everything is looser and softer; therefore it is very important that pregnant women don't work terribly hard to increase their stretch. They should work to feel the stretch as we do in Yoga, but they should be encouraged not to push themselves too far. A strong, intermediate student might want to work hard, but she must not overstretch. Moreover because the hormone relaxin remains in the system for 3 months after you have given birth, especially if nursing, you should be careful not to overstretch during the whole time.

Lilias: What would you recommend to a beginner and to a student who has been studying Hatha Yoga?

Judith: The student of a few months is much the same as a beginner, except that there is a little more awareness of what Hatha Yoga is. The greatest benefits of Yoga in childbirth are not only the physical, but also the mental effects Hatha Yoga produces. It's not only learning how to relax, but also learning to accept what comes to you; these are the keys to a good birth experience, and to raising a baby, too. One of the most important things is the relaxation practice at the end of class. It's a beautiful way of letting go, and that's the key in labor if you want to give birth naturally.

Lilias: For a woman who has never done Hatha Yoga, is it safe to start when she's 2 months pregnant?

Judith: I think Yoga is probably one of the best all-around systems for helping someone enjoy the pregnancy and go through it healthily and happily. There is no physiological reason why, after a woman (rank beginner) has checked with her doctor and has received an okay, that she shouldn't or couldn't do Twists, Forward Bends, or modified Shoulder-stands. The intermediate student can do other postures. The only poses you should be careful with are the backbends or lying on the back too long, or anything that overstretches the abdomen, after the first 3 to 4 months, because the softening of the tissues can cause small herniations of the abdominal muscles.

For example, after 3½ to 4 months, I did the Camel and I felt a very strong tugging at the breastbone, where the abdominal muscles are attached. This told me there was too much stress on them, so I gave up backbends. There is no physiological reason why you cannot lie on your stomach and do the Bow, if it feels good to you. *The whole key is to do what feels good to you.*

A pregnant woman is much more in tune to what is happening within her body than at any other time in her life. The problem is that most pregnant women haven't done any physical activities, and then, about six months along, feel that they should do something

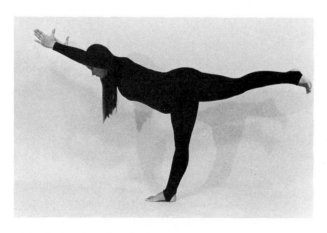

"The key is do what feels good to you." Judith Lasater, eight months pregnant.

for their bodies, so they take a 6-week course in child-birth. To me, that's not enough to let you get into the way of thinking about your breathing, your mind states, your energy, your body tone, and how they all fit together. For all of these, Yoga is great! I accept people in my classes all the way along anytime they want to start, and I have gotten great feedback on how valuable Hatha Yoga has been to them.

It's also fantastic in the post-partum stage. As soon as you feel like it, you can start Yoga after childbirth. The first thing you would begin with is a simple Forward Bend, sitting down. This doesn't take a lot of strength or energy. Even though I had a surgical delivery, I began Yoga on the eighth day after birth. You can then add simple twists. These are good to tone the abdomen and to get it back into shape. Then add a few simple standing poses, then a few beginning back arches. The *last* thing you add are inverted poses. You need to wait at least 4 to 6 weeks until the lochia has stopped completely. (This is the bleeding flow after birth, caused by the uterus healing from inside, where the placenta has been torn away.) Inverted poses started too early can cause bleeding again.

Lilias: What other exercises did you find important and would recommend?

Judith: I swam. Swimming and walking are so important! Swimming is wonderful because, instead of feeling big and awkward, you feel light and graceful. It was very cosmic, thinking of the baby floating in me and me floating in the water.

And I walked. Walking helps circulation and the mind. I jogged for a while, but only so long as it felt comfortable. My pace got slower and slower, and then I walked. I found I couldn't run very well because my diaphragm couldn't descend, and I couldn't breathe deeply enough because the baby was in the way. Therefore I had to slow down. I did continue swimming; I did it for my endurance. I couldn't swim fast, but I did improve my distance.

I find endurance is basically a mental phenomenon. If I know I've run 3 miles, I feel it shows me what inner strength I have. Walking, swimming and other such exercises, combined with Yoga, can be beneficial for pregnant women.

Lilias: Do you have other helpful hints that made you feel more comfortable mentally or physically?

Judith: One of the best poses was getting on all fours, lifting my back up and slowly dropping down to a slight arch. This brings the uterus back into position. It also is great in relieving back strain. I did this several times a day about 10 to 15 repetitions each time.

The squat position is also good. Actually when

you squat, you open the pelvis up to an inch. Many women in other cultures deliver in this position. It's a good position for pregnant women, so long as you make sure your feet are parallel and that your feet don't turn out, which puts a strain on the inner knee. The squat also relieves back pressures. It is a good way to go to the bathroom if you are having constipation.

Lilias: What are pelvic-floor exercises?

Judith: Pelvic-floor exercises are good and easy to do. These are also called Kegal exercises or Kegals. (Kegal is a physician who wrote a book called *Key To Feminine Response in Marriage*.) Basically, the Kegal is the same thing the ancients called *Aswini Mudra*, a contraction of the anal and vaginal areas of the pelvic floor.

Aswini Mudra is very important for all women to learn, especially during pregnancy. To do one, simply contract the vagina and hold for a count of 5, then release to a count of 5, working up to 10. Then contract the anus and repeat the counting. This movement is helpful during crowning of the baby's head (the last stages of birth) because the conscious relaxation of the pelvic floor allows the baby's head to come through the vagina. If you strengthen this area, it is easier to relax it and allow the tissues to stretch. You can do these sitting, in the car while waiting at stop lights, or while listening to music.

Lilias: Is it complicated to do or to feel this?

Judith: You're really concentrating on the vaginal area, but you can't really separate the two (anus and vagina). If people can't feel what it feels like, tell them to contract the anus very hard; they'll feel the vagina contracting. This is supposed to get the pelvic floor in condition. This exercise has the added benefit of helping to prevent urinating when one coughs or sneezes. This exercise is great for all women. It helps them control these muscles during the sexual act, and in reaching orgasm.

One other thing I wanted to mention is creative visualization during Savasana [Relaxation]. During relaxation, I have my students visualize the cervix, a long, narrow, necklike end of the uterus that leads to the vagina. Then, during the last few weeks of pregnancy, during relaxation, I have them visualize the cervix softening, which it does near the end of pregnancy and in labor. A woman who visualizes the softening of her cervix can speed up the labor process.

I have a friend who teaches prenatal Yoga classes in California. She has had such success that the hospital where most of her students go to give birth is doing a study on it, because her students give birth so fast. They want to find out if it's the Yoga or the visualization or both. Many of her students give birth in 2, 3, or 4 hours as compared to 9, 10, or 12 hours for a first birth.

You would not want to do visualization in the early stages of pregnancy. We would suggest using it 6 weeks before and during labor. Then it would be physiologically safe because this is what's going to be happening naturally.

Lilias: I knew nothing about natural childbirth 18 years ago and fought the contractions every inch of the way.

Judith: When you have a contraction, the tendency is to run away from it, and Yoga teaches us that running away from pain is what has got us into this uncomfortable condition of being so tight in our muscles, so unhappy in our minds. Yoga is recognizing, surrendering, and then letting go of pain, experiencing discomfort, tenseness and tightness you carry with you and then letting it out; Yoga lets you get rid of it. Labor is uncomfortable, but by visualizing what is happening and letting go to help the body give birth, one can make birth a more fulfilling experience.

Lilias: What cautions would you give women who wish to start Yoga during their pregnancy?

Judith: Even if you do have problems, you can adapt and do *some* form of Yoga. The only caution I would offer for anyone pregnant doing Yoga would be to one having "cervical insufficiency." This is rare. It means that the cervix doesn't stay tight, and many times women with this problem miscarry. There is a procedure to rectify this. However, I would discourage anyone with this from doing Yoga.

Lilias: Tell me briefly about your own delivery.

Judith: We wanted to have our child, Miles, at home for a variety of reasons. We were healthy and prepared mentally and physically. I'm a trained Bradley childbirth instructor, and a physical therapist. With these qualifications and a daily practice of Yoga, we felt we could manage a home birth successfully. We had visited the hospital, and so we had a backup if needed. I also had a midwife.

I went into labor. It appeared that it was going to be very slow. I accepted this and said, "I know, but we're really going to make it!" It went on for a really long time. I got up to 7 centimeters (you must be up to 10 centimeters to deliver), and then it seemed it wasn't getting anywhere. I had been in labor nearly two days, and I was getting exhausted, so we went to the hospital. After a few hours in the hospital, I had an X-ray and it was found that I had cephalic pelvic disproportion, i.e., the baby's head and my pelvis were disproportionate. The doctor said they'd have to do a caesarian section.

At the mention of caesarian everything seemed to stop. I found myself within a vision, a time

Yoga and Pregnancy

warp. I saw two paths. I was faced with going down the right-hand path or the left. On the left-hand path, I was freaking out; I was getting angry, creating a terrible vibration for myself, my baby, my husband, and for the people present. I was into a real "me" against "them" thing. "Why are they doing this to me?" On the right-hand path, calmness was being presented to me. "Fine, thus and thus is what is happening to me. It's my karma, my lesson. I can accept it. I can *choose* to make it as loving and as freeing an experience as I wish." It was like a split second of time; everything stopped. Because of my Yoga training, that constant observation, I chose consciously to walk on the right-hand path, and I'm so grateful I did because I could have gone either way. I said to myself, okay, and I suddenly felt an incredible inner strength.

It was difficult. I didn't want this situation. I don't even like to take an aspirin. I wanted a home birth: here I was having a complicated birth. I, a Yoga teacher! I feel it was because of my decision from the real inner strength I had been given, that Miles and I did so well. I was able to go home 3 days later and was jogging in 3 weeks. It was wonderful!

Lilias: I know what you mean by being the observer, and that one does have free will and choices.

Judith: That was what Yoga did for me in my first birth experience. It was so important for me to learn that *I can't control everything!* When we get into Yoga, we think "If I eat these foods, do these poses, think such and such thoughts, then I can control what happens to me." I'm learning that you cannot control what happens to you, but you can control *your response* to what happens to you. What's important is how you respond to a death, an illness, or whatever life deals to you. That's the key that Yoga gives us; you have a *choice* in how you respond.

Lilias: How about after the birth?

Judith: I was a little depressed when I went home because I had been unable to deliver naturally at home. I ate a lot of alfalfa and drank a lot of comfrey tea; I started breast feeding. That helped a lot. Birth is just a matter of hours, and then there is the nursing and the raising of the baby. You can divorce a husband, but you can't divorce your child: there's always that permanent bond. I decided when I got home that I was not going to feel like a failure, and that I was not going to let my disappointment ruin my life and my relationship with my baby. Yoga helped me mentally. It seemed to affect the hospital, too. They broke all sorts of rules. My husband Ike and Miles our new son were brought into the recovery room; they let us all stay together.

Lilias: It sounds as if a higher power gave you an experience far beyond what you had pictured for yourself and your home delivery.

Judith: It did. Everyone, including me, had such great expectations. I can see now how those expectations can be false and misleading. It is very freeing to find out you're human; you don't have to live up to that perfect Yoga-teacher image.

Interview with an Obstetrician

When my children were young, I can remember reading *Birth Without Violence* by Dr. Frederick Leboyer. I was pleased and deeply grateful when some years later, life's dance brought the two of us together for a television interview.

If you have not read *Birth Without Violence*, please do. The book's gentle, enlightened text about birth and life are for everyone, male and female. The incredible photographs of the first few moments in the new baby's life, as it is introduced lovingly, quietly, tenderly, and thoughtfully to its new surroundings, are a joy to behold.

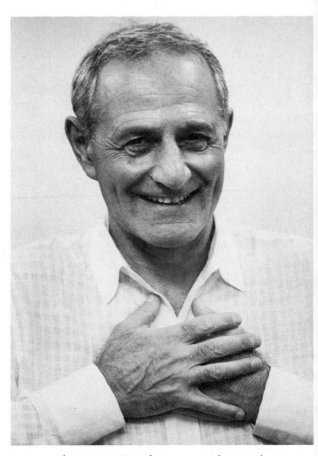

It is my pleasure to introduce you to this gentle warrior, Frederick Leboyer

Lilias, Yoga, and Your Life

Meeting Dr. Leboyer was a highlight of my life.

Leboyer: Usually when a child is born, people examine it carefully, and when they are satisfied the baby is all right, they put it aside and are finished. And a few days later the baby is taken home.

I work differently. Because a baby is very sensitive, I talk to it. "Do you mind if I touch you? May I touch you? Oh! Yes. You are beautiful! If you don't mind I want to check a few things. Yes. I can see you are perfectly all right. I am very happy with you. Thank you."

Unfortunately, most people don't talk to newborn babies. The baby is checked as one checks a machine, rather than as somebody who is very aware of what is going on and is terrified and, moreover, infuriated and humiliated not to be understood as already being somebody.

Imagine that you are completely paralyzed. I think you're dead, and you have time to make me understand you are not dead, but you have only your eyes to do so. If suddenly I touch your eyes, you see that I see; you know that I have understood. You are relieved.

The baby is trying to make people understand. It doesn't talk, of course, but it's expressing that it doesn't very much like the way it's being treated. It is suffering in its heart, not in its body, infuriated not to be understood for what it is. That's all there is to it.

If people then fail to understand this point, they have a tendency to turn it into a technique and talk of the Leboyer technique. No.

Lilias: It starts with the heart. You established comunication, so there was union. And that's what Yoga really is.

Leboyer: Yes, but one must be very careful with the words *heart* and *love*; my approach is not emotional. Nor is it sentimental. No. Even if people want to see it like this, a warm, loving, emotional experience, it is far better to do this than to see the newborn baby as a *something*. It's underway then, and when you're underway, you progress from an understanding that becomes deeper and deeper and deeper. You progress continually.

Lilias: You have a very special way of talking about and writing about a woman who is pregnant. Many women feel heavy, ungainly. It's a difficult time, especially at 8 or 9 months. You must see something. Can you explain what you see?

Leboyer: It's hard to explain. It's so great, so extraordinary to be expecting a baby. It's not a disease. It's got nothing to do with health; nothing to do with the medical profession in any way. Yes, when something really goes wrong, one *must* have the help of a skilled, knowledgeable obstetrician. I'm not denying this at all, but I would say there's more to being pregnant than the medical eye can see.

Lilias: What about the pain in childbirth and the pain in performing the Asanas?

Leboyer: The fear of pain in birth is closely connected to the fear of pain in Asana. There is pain when you are afraid of something and because you're afraid of it, you try to reject it, fight it. When there is pain or fear, it means you're trying to run away from something, and if you want to understand anything, first you must be with it. The natural tendency is to fight it as soon as it appears. This is so not only for Yoga, but also for much of the so-called Western way of life. As soon as it hurts, we use some technique to get rid of it. The only true attitude regarding physical, mental, or any type of pain is simply to accept it fully. Open to it and taste it. Do not run away from it; do not fight it in order to punish yourself. There is no sin, no guilty feeling. One must only get fully a taste of it, and if you open fully to it, instead of running away from it or trying to stop it, something happens. You're dancing to something else, some understanding, some knowledge.

Lilias: In a sense it becomes your teacher.

Leboyer: Yes. But let's not put any qualification on it; otherwise, we start building expectation, and whenever we expect, we cannot help being frustrated. Any expectation is bound to meet frustration because it's a projection of the past. We experienced something that was enjoyable, and we want to experience it again. The truth is that everything is new, new, new, new, continuously from moment to moment. Nothing is ever going to be as we expect it, even an Asana. It is always new. Why? Because you get deeper and deeper into it. Your understanding and your experience widen and get deeper and deeper. It's always the same, always, and yet it's always not.

Lilias: Do you recommend that pregnant women do Asanas?

Leboyer: No. Certainly not. If they want to, they are most welcome, but I am not trying to say that this is the way.

Lilias: In your book, *Inner Beauty, Inner Light*, you have a wonderful model, I believe the second daughter of B. K. S. Iyengar, doing a beautiful Asana, the Shoulderstand, using a chair as an aid.

Leboyer: The chair is not an aid, but a lead, a teacher, just as when the wall is used.

Lilias: Are there certain postures you wouldn't recommend for the pregnant woman?

Leboyer: Lying flat on the stomach is not advisable. Any other posture, with some limitations, is all right, and limitations would come from your pure and proper understanding of the aim and significance of the posture. These postures should be done under the supervision of a teacher because one must check moment by moment exactly what is going on. During pregnancy, one must be exceptionally careful. This is the most important restriction that Yoga should be done always under the personal guidance of a teacher.

Lilias: Have you studied with Mr. Iyengar?

Leboyer: Yes. I had been doing Yoga for quite a while before I met Mr. Iyengar in Poona, India.

Lilias: What does Yoga mean to you?

Leboyer: Not to run away. To be fully with an experience, and not to panic when it begins to become uncomfortable. To be bold enough and have enough to get the taste of it. If you don't run away, if you don't fight back, something happens, and you get to learn about yourself, first, and, second, you get to learn about your breathing. Don't try to conduct it, or guide it. No. Open to your own breathing. Your breathing becomes your teacher. Don't try to use it; be used by your own breathing, as it were. Open up, open up and flow.

Interview with a New Mother

Joannie Surber, 22, did her poses up until three weeks before the baby arrived. He was named Jacob Aaron. I asked her about her practice during pregnancy.

Joannie: I did my Yoga stretching and breathing all the way through. Carrying the extra weight low on my back, I found that the Forward Bend and the Side Bow felt especially good to me, since they relieved the aching pressure in my lower back.

Yoga relaxation is so special and different because you learn to go through control and release of all the different muscles at will. It was a more in-depth relaxation than in my natural childbirth classes. Because I was trained in this sort of awareness, I stayed very much in touch with what was happening all through my home delivery.

My doctor said I was the first woman who stopped pushing before he said to stop pushing. I could just *feel* when the muscles were stretched and when they weren't.

Now my stomach muscles are coming back slowly, but I'm back to my same dress size as before. I think it was the Yoga that kept my *shape*, even though I gained a little extra weight. Everything stayed firm. I didn't go soft and blubbery!

A DAILY SCHEDULE

The following practice schedule is a gentle and safe start for the pregnant beginning Yoga student. It is best to begin as soon as you know you are pregnant, although you can start any time during pregnancy. If you do not have a formal teacher, I suggest you read the directions carefully and proceed slowly doing the exercises in the order given for about 20 minutes each day. Always conclude with the three steps of Relaxation.

Do not attempt the more advanced postures in other sections without the guidance of a formal teacher. *Be sure* to avoid the following poses:

1. Stomach Lift
2. Leg Raises, as they might cause abdominal or back strain late in pregnancy. Or, if you prefer, Leg Raises with Bent Knee until your abdomen becomes uncomfortable.
3. Locust. The Locust gives you a strong contraction of the uterus. It is to be avoided throughout pregnancy.

BEGINNER'S PRACTICE SCHEDULE
(Time duration 20 minutes)

Pelvic Tilt
Table
Cat Stretch
Dog Wag
Pose of a Child
Squat
Relax in Sponge. Take 6 Complete Breaths
Forward Bend (with aid of towel)
Groin Stretch
Sitting Twist (with blanket)
Legs Apart in V with Forward Bend
Side Bow (only if comfortable)
Half Shoulderstand
Rest with legs on a chair, 1–3 minutes
Sponge—5 minutes

KEGAL'S (ASWINI MUDRA)

This is a great exercise for women of all ages!

The perineal floor is a muscular sling that extends from the pubic bone to the rectum. This musle sling provides support for the pelvic organs. These organs are the urethra, vagina and the rectum. These muscles stretch considerably for birth. After he birth, it is important they return to their job providing support to the pelvic organs. To maintain good muscle tone and flexibility before and after pregnancy, do the following exercises. It has the added benefit of helping to prevent urinating when one coughs or sneezes.

1. Sit on the edge of a chair, knees apart, feet flat on the floor. Inhale and tighten your sphincter muscle and entire pelvic floor will tighten. Hold to count of 5.
Exhale and push down to press pelvic floor toward chair.
2. Sit cross-legged and repeat Number 1.
3. Stop and start urine flow 5 times when urinating.
4. After the techniques in Numbers 1 to 3 are strong and comfortable, do pelvic floor exercises 1 or 2 times every waking hour.

TABLE

A foundation pose to build the Cat Stretch and Dog Wag poses.
Kneel on a mat. Your spine is straight as a table and stomach pulled in. Hands are on mat directly parallel to shoulders. Elbows are straight, fingertips facing forward, knees on either side of stomach. Knees should be lined up with hips.

CAT STRETCH

Excellent stimulation of the nerves within the spine. Gentle massage of inner organs. Aids in constipation and digestion.
Assume Table pose.
Exhale, round spine, tighten sphincter muscle and bring chin gently to throat.
Inhale, chin up to ceiling. Concave lower spine, tailbone up toward ceiling.
Repeat this motion 4 to 8 times slowly and smoothly. Be attentive to breathing.

Variation

As you inhale and lift chin, lift right leg up toward ceiling.
Repeat one to three times each leg.
After you do either of the above poses, rest in Pose of a Child.

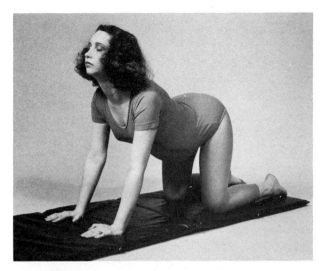

Cat Stretch

POSE OF A CHILD

A wonderful pose to rest and relax in. Soothes lower back. Opens up the pelvis and gives extra circulation to the nerves of the lower spine.
Kneel so that knees are on either side of stomach, comfortably apart so you can breathe easily.
Placing forehead on the floor, or turning cheek to floor, put arms alongside legs, hands opposite feet.
Relax shoulders, neck and arms. Breathe comfortably.
Rest for a few minutes.

FORWARD BEND

Increases blood circulation to the entire spine, aids in flexibility in pelvis and hips, and stretches the back of legs. Helps you relax *during* tension. Relaxes the muscles that talk back to you with words of stiffness! This process is helpful training in preparing you to learn how to relax during contractions.
Sit on the edge of a folded mat so that your sitting bones are elevated. (This will help overcome stiffness in your hips.)
Place towel behind feet, and if your stomach is big, place your legs in a V.
Grab the towel behind your feet and inhale. Then exhale your upper body toward your thighs.
Hold the position as long as you like, while breathing comfortably. Relax your neck, face, shoulders, hands, arms, the backs of your thighs and buttocks. Release the tightness in all these muscles.
When you are done, release slowly, lie down and relax. Observe how the pose has affected your body.

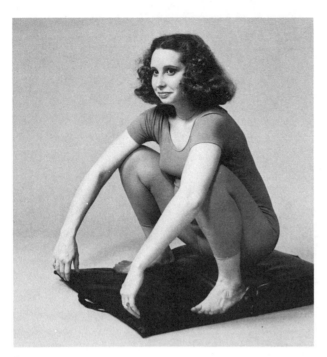

Squat

SQUAT

Relieves back pressure. Aids constipation problems. Opens up the pelvic area. Increases circulation to pelvic area.

Raise your heels and place them on a folded mat, blanket, or book. Stand with feet pointed *straight* ahead 12 inches apart (hip distance). Anything farther than hip distance causes strain on knee cartilage.

Squat comfortably for as long as you like on the back of your heels, arms resting comfortably on knees.

Easy to do totally clothed and while watching TV.

SEATED GROIN STRETCH

This exercise stretches the ligaments and muscles of the inner thigh and increases the flexibility of the hips and the entire pelvic area.

Sit on the edge of a folded blanket.

Place the soles of the feet together. Open knees.

Pressing the soles of the feet together with your hands, try to lift the upper part of the feet.

Gently pulling head back, inhale while lifting chest and relaxing the neck.

As you hold smoothly, inhaling and exhaling, your inner thigh muscles will relax.

Each time you lift your head, inhale. Let the chest open, and the deep abdominal breathing will happen spontaneously.

Hold as long as you like, surrendering to the stretch of the Asana, and the knees will come down effortlessly.

Variation

Lie down, buttocks against the wall, knees bent, feet together, heels close to groin.

Place your hands on your knees. Inhale; then, exhaling, press knees gently toward the wall. Inhale again. Release slightly, then exhaling, repeat above.

SEATED SIDE TWIST

Your hips will remain straight ahead as you do the Spinal Twist. Enjoy the pleasant easing up feeling within the spine as you do this pose.

Fold a blanket or place a pillow beneath right buttock only.

Bend the knees, draw the right foot in close to your left thigh, knees apart on the floor, left foot behind you.

Place your right hand on floor, where it falls naturally, fingers pointed to your right and *away* from your body.

Place the fingers of your left hand under your right knee.

Straighten your arms. Exhaling and lifting yourself, gently press the fingertips into the floor. This

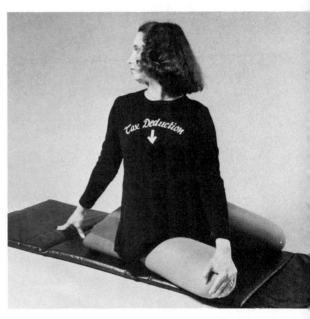

Seated Side Twist

simple stretching movement of your arms will turn your torso to the right. First, turn shoulder to right followed by the chin, nose, and eyes.

Unwind the pose slowly, releasing and relaxing the eyes, neck, shoulders, and rib cage as you go. Repeat once more.

Change leg position and repeat twice on opposite side.

FORWARD BEND, LEGS IN V

If you were not pregnant I would instruct you to bring your forehead to the floor in this exercise. Given your special condition, I recommend you simply try to achieve a good sitting posture and start the forward motion.

Stretches and tones the inner thighs, hip, and pelvic area.

Sit close to the edge of folded blanket on your sitting bones.

Place your legs wide enough apart so that you feel the stretch but are still comfortable.

Relax the shoulders and rest hands lightly on legs.

Inhale, lifting the sternum and, exhaling, slowly bring stomach forward as if to rest upon the ground. This breathing should be as effortless as your heartbeat. Try to be aware of the breath and body moving as one.

Note how the back seems to open with each spontaneous and deep breath.

Hold for 30 seconds, working up to one minute. Relax your face, shoulders, and arms.

Release. Bring legs together and shake your knees out.

Close your eyes, observe how the legs feel, lie down, in Sponge pose, and take three complete breaths.

SIDE BOW

Joannie enjoyed doing this more vigorous stretch for spine and abdomen, even being eight months along, because it made her feel so good. However, you should do this movement only if you enjoy it.

Lie on right side. Reach back and clasp your ankles, right hand to right ankle; left hand to left.

Inhale; gently squeeze shoulder blades together. Lift the ankles. Lift the chin.

Hold a few seconds, breathing comfortably, feeling the stretch. Release; then turn over to the opposite side.

Repeat Side Bow on left side.

Rest deeply in the Pose of a Child, knees bent with feet apart on either side of your stomach.

SPONGE (RELAXATION POSE)

This conscious relaxation quiets the restless mind, recharges batteries, and can be applied to your natural childbirth classes.

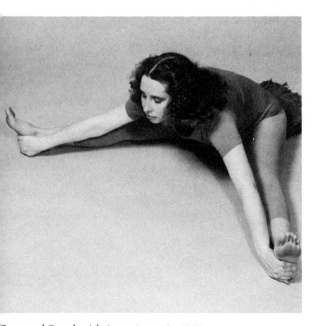

Forward Bend with Legs Apart in "V"

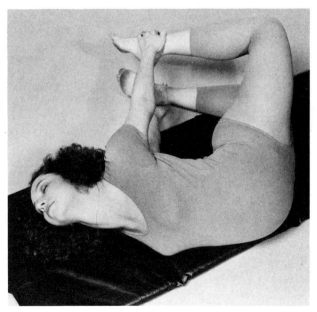

Side Bow

It is best not to lie flat on your back for long periods of time as it is uncomfortable for your back. When you do choose to rest this way, arrange a pillow so that your head and chest are supported, and place one beneath your knees to relieve tightness in your lower back.

Then spend 5 or 10 minutes relaxing your body. Reread and use the three steps of Relaxation (from chapter 3). Focus on each part of the body, starting with your toes and working up to the top of your head. Suggest to that part of the body to relax; then pause and feel the sensation of relaxation.

You might find some of the simple tension relievers from page 84 helpful for release of physical or emotional tension.

Lying on your side is perfect for relaxation, especially in the last weeks of pregnancy and during labor. Place your body carefully, and with awareness, into this pose. Notice that when in this pose, the body forms a Swastika, the ancient symbol for the whirling, circulating movement of life's energy.

SWASTIKA

Lie on your right side. Right arm is behind you, elbow bent, palm facing the ceiling. Left hand is in front of you, elbow bent, palm down to the floor.

Bend your left knee close to your left elbow so the thigh forms right angle to the body and the calf makes a right angle to the thigh.

As you come near the end of your pregnancy, place a pillow beneath the left knee for support. This will effortlessly open the pelvis.

Exhale, as if heaving a sigh of happiness and well-being. Surrender all tensions, fears, and doubts. As

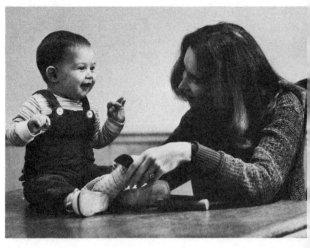

Introducing Jacob Aaron Suber

you empty your chest, the natural weight of your body will accentuate the twist in the spine and bring the left shoulder closer to the floor.

After relaxing on your right side, turn over and relax on the left.

DAILY ROUTINE BEFORE CHILDBIRTH

First Week

Pelvic Tilt
Dog Wag
Off-the-Wall exercises
Cat Stretch
Pose of a Child
Squat
Relax in Sponge—take 6 Complete Breaths
Windmill
Side Leg Lifts
Relax in Sponge for 5 minutes

Second Week

Repeat all exercises from first week.
Working on Picking Apples and the Hulk from "All
    Shoulder Work" section.
Relax in Sponge—take 6 Complete Breaths
Forward Bend
Seated Groin Stretch
Seated Side Twist
Bridge
Star
Complete Breath and 5-minute Relaxation Sponge

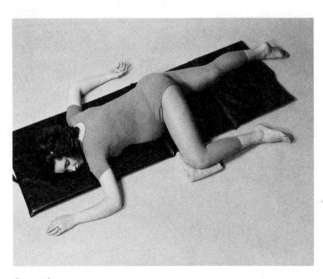

Swastika

Lilias, Yoga, and Your Life

Third Week

Any two tension relievers
Repeat your favorite from the first week.
Relax in Sponge—Take 6 Complete Breaths
Forward Bend with Legs Apart in a V
Lunge with a Chair
Side Bow (if comfortable)
Half Shoulderstand (if comfortable)
6 Complete Breaths and 5-minute Sponge, using the
    Swastika pose.

ROUTINE AFTER CHILDBIRTH

After childbirth, and with your doctor's okay, do
the following exercises in the order given:

First Week

Rock-a-Baby (no pun intended)
One Leg Forward Bend with Towel
Forward Bend
Forward Bend with Legs in V
Complete Breath and Sponge

Second Week

Repeat first week's exercises
Seated Side Twist
One Leg Forward Bend with Twist
6 Complete Breaths and 5 minute Sponge

Third Week

All of first week's exercises
All of second week's exercises
Relax in Sponge—Take 6 Complete Breaths
Easy Rock and Roll
Knees Side to Side
Twist in a Chair

Easy Twist
6 Complete Breaths and 5 minute Sponge

Fourth Week

Any tension reliever
Knees Side to Side
One Leg Forward Bend with Towel
Off-the-Wall exercises
Bridge 1 and 2
Relax in Sponge—take 6 Complete Breaths
Windmill
Do 2 of your favorite leg exercises
Fish Over a Barrel
Spinal Warmups 1, 2 and 3
Chest Expander
6 Complete Breaths and Sponge for 5 minutes.

Eight to Twelve Weeks

After all discharge has stopped, you may add
inverted poses such as the Shoulderstand.

EXERCISES DURING MENSTRUATION

I am often asked by women who are not pregnant, "Should I exercise during my menstrual cycle?"
My own feeling is, *listen* to your body. If some postures such as the Inverted Pose or Locust bring on a
heavy flow, then avoid them. Do other poses that
are gentle to the abdominal area. The effect of these
postures is different for each woman. Most doctors
do not object to your exercising during your period;
they feel that exercises reduce menstrual cramps and
tension.

Be cautious if you wear an IUD. Avoid poses
such as Stomach Lift and the Locust. Some women,
however, have never displaced their IUD and have
practiced Yoga for years.

Listen and be aware of your own body and how
it functions, and you'll do fine!

18

Hatha Yoga Exercises for Preschool Children

"Should I teach Yoga exercises to my child?" This question is often asked by students all over the country who have received so many benefits themselves and wish to share them with their children. Yes, Hatha Yoga can be a wonderful experience for children. However, one of the biggest problems is finding a weekly class for youngsters of all different ages. Little by little, nursery schools, grade schools, and junior and senior high schools are bringing aspects of Yoga into their daily exercise programs. Physical educators are seeing the merits of the slow movements, breathing and relaxation.

Teaching a child, age six on up, is definitely different from working with a child of two and a half to five. A Yoga class for the child of six or older can be approached very similarly to an adult class. In this age group, I recommend a balanced half-hour program of Yoga poses from the chapter on simple breathing techniques, and a shorthand version of relaxation. *Balanced* means using postures that encourage the spine to move forward, backward, side to side, and in a twist motion. It also means finding individual poses that encourage balancing, flexibility, and strength. As a teacher, you'd vary this half-hour program each time. Using the English names instead of the Sanskrit will make the exercise more understandable and will stimulate the children's creativity and imagination.

Sometimes the pace of an adult class is just *too* slow for the older child (ages 6 or up) and causes restlessness. However, if the temperament and concentration level are such that the older child is still interested in joining an adult class, then try it out. I have seen it work, especially if the mother, or father and child share and experience it together. What a lovely link to have in common!

My only strong feelings about teaching Yoga to children is *not to teach the Headstand or High Shoulderstand*. It can be extremely injurious to the muscles of the upper neck and to the alignment of the delicate vertebrae of the young neck. This pose, in particular, is not to be taken lightly or as a game for a child, or for that matter, for an adult!

Interview with a Preschool Teacher

Working with the preschooler from ages 2½ up to 5 is another matter. Recently, I went to my first preschool Yoga class held at the Jewish Community Center of Cincinnati, Ohio. What I found was truly beautiful. Suzie Schreiber has been teaching these classes since 1974. I noticed many things about her class that were different. Later, we talked about these and other challenges.

Lilias: Is there any difference between teaching Yoga to 2-to-3-year-olds and 4-to-5-year-olds.

Suzie: The length of the class time is the same for both age groups. However, the younger children have a *very* short attention span. I have to go from exercise to exercise relatively quickly. The Quiet Place relaxation has to be shorter, maybe 5 to 10

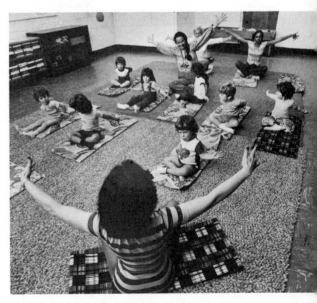

Suzie Schreiber with Class

seconds. I also have to make some of the exercises a little bit sillier by using childish names for poses such as Prune Face or Sleepy-Foot-Baby. Using different voice inflections and babyish words such as Wiggly Toes instead of Move Your Toes, does make it more fun and keeps their attention on me; otherwise, they will drift.

Lilias: What about working with the 4- and 5-year-olds?

Suzie: The older children enjoy the silly faces and some of the silly words, but they don't *need* them. I can be more adult, and still make it fun. When we do Sleepy-Foot-Baby, and some of the 'macho' boys resist, I'll tell them, "This is a very important exercise for the muscle at the top of your leg and your hips. It helps you to run fast. It helps you to jump high." Then, I say, "If you just hold your leg, you don't have to pretend that it's a baby. You are stretching that muscle by rolling it back and forth."

The attention span of this age is longer, and I can give more rest between exercises. Their Quiet Place relaxation can go longer than half a minute. The class is still kept to 15 to 20 minutes.

Lilias: What are some of the difficulties in teaching preschool children?

Suzie: Some days Yoga goes smoothly. They all listen. It goes beautifully. Other days, they're all wound up; there's been a lot of snow or rain; they haven't been outside, or there's that special electricity in the air. It is then that the teacher needs to sit down quietly with the children and to get in touch with what sort of mood they're in so she feels intuitively what needs to be done. If they're wound up, I'll get up and do an active exercise where we can all feel the heart beat. More active exercises help to slow them down and allow their energy to dissipate itself. I don't know how or why we have few disciplinary problems, or why the kids don't wander around. Perhaps having their own individual mat gives them a feeling of their own comfortable and secure place. They also know it's a quiet time. Their voices have to be quiet, so they can hear mine.

Lilias: What do you do when some children don't want to exercise that day?

Suzie: I find that very easy. I just ask them to rest on their mats, saying, "You don't have to do Yoga today." They usually enjoy watching and then will join in without being forced.

Lilias: What about the talking or giggling?

Suzie: I ignore it; soon they calm down and start listening to what comes next. For the most part, I'll put my fingers to my lips; the children will stop because they are usually looking at me. They test you. They'll talk, knowing you don't want them to; soon

they stop, realizing that it doesn't bother me. I don't ever let it get out of hand. Every now and then there'll be a slight behavior problem. Very, very seldom have I needed to remove a child from Yoga class.

Lilias: Do you have adult helpers in your Yoga classes?

Suzie: Only one teacher or sometimes one parent; some have previous Yoga experience; others do not. I encourage and feel it is *important* that the helper participate in all exercises and not just sit there and watch. If children of this age see a teacher or helper not doing the exercise, they'll not do it. "Monkey see, Monkey do." The helper can aid me by occasionally quietly walking around to a child and encouraging him or her into a pose, or by just watching.

Lilias: Do you ever help children into a pose?

Suzie: I rarely have to help them into a pose. I do not feel the poses need to be perfect! When a young child puts himself or herself comfortably into a pose, *that* is the safe and correct positioning for his or her own body. When they imitate what I do, they will keep themselves in check and will not allow things to become strenuous.

The only pose that I aid in is the Bow. When they are lying on their stomach, trying to find their ankles with their hands, and to figure out how to lift up their heads, then I help. I'll put my hand under the chest (not ever touching the neck!) and lift gently, so that the child can feel that the lift comes from underneath part of the body, rather than from the neck muscles. This is when the assistant can also help easily and safely, so that there is no worry of overstraining.

Lilias: Do the children have to wear anything special? And how about the room?

Suzie: Clothing? They can wear anything. They should have a soft mat, towel or blanket or something soft that is their own space; then they control themselves. The carpet is lovely, but does not allow them their own space.

I encourage them to take their shoes off because it's the only way they can really wiggle their toes and have their feet get fresh air, and move their ankles. If a child is inhibited, I don't insist, but do tell them to keep their feet off the mat, so that the mat stays clean. After a while, they'll take their shoes off.

If it's a nice day, I prefer to have no artificial lighting. I open the shades to let the sunlight in. It's more peaceful.

Lilias: How would you lead a preschool child into a Quiet Place of Relaxation What are the words you use?

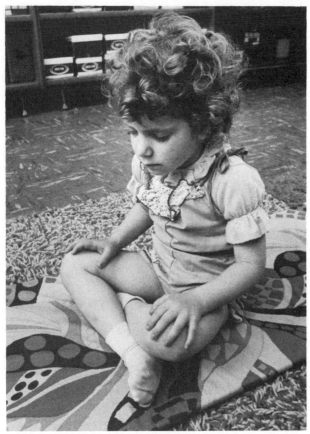

Be very very still and go into your quiet place.

Suzie: I say, in a soft voice:

Take your hands and put them in your lap. (Some children like to lie down in their Quiet Place, so they lie down.)

Be very, very still. This is a chance for your body to have a rest from all the things it has done today. This is a time to get some new energy and just to turn everything off.

With hands in your lap, close your eyes.

Turn off all parts of your body factory.

Turn off the wiggles in your toes.

Turn off the wiggles in your hands.

Let your back, stomach, legs, and arms rest.

Turn off everything in your body factory except for your breathing, and that goes in and out by itself.

It's a chance for your ears to exercise and listen to everything that's going on around us.

Now, be very, very still.

Lilias: What fascinated me during that brief relaxation was that I could hear and feel a difference in vibration within the room. They really did go to a quiet place. What a wonderful tool to give a child at such an early age. They can have control over their emotions and actions.

Suzie: Yes, I've seen a child wound up or crying, or afraid, on the playground, or in classes and then I watched a nursery-teacher who is familiar with the Quiet-Place technique, help the child to concentrate on counting the breath in and out and on relaxing body parts. I've tried it with children who have been really crying; it works beautifully! Life is hectic now even for children. They can learn Yoga now, they can slow down and be aware of their bodies and exercise restfully. They can control their muscles and emotions in tight situations. Learning Hatha Yoga when you are very young will carry over into adulthood, especially if their mothers and fathers are also practicing some form of Yoga and can give the child support.

Lilias: What a head start! Fantastic!

PREFACE TO EXERCISE PROGRAM

Here are three, short, 15-minute Yoga exercise programs written (with Suzie Schreiber's guidance) especially for nursery-school children. I have written them as I would give them in a class. If you or your child find the words babyish, or you enjoy using the Sanskrit names, change the wording to suit your needs.

These exercises can be adapted for the retarded child or the child with motor-ability difficulties; they have been extremely helpful in working with the hyperactive youngster. They also could be used as an alternative exercise program for the severely retarded adult. These exercises can be taught by a

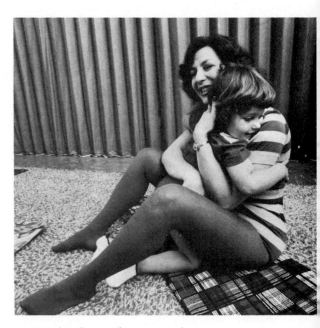

Suzie Schreiber with Young Admirer

Lilias, Yoga, and Your Life

loving parent, or a caring teacher who has had previous experience in Hatha Yoga other than book information (although it's not totally necessary). There is nothing like sharing what you know and have learned, because you've *experienced* it yourself.

PROGRAM FOR PRESCHOOL CHILDREN (2½–5)

Most of these foot-and-face exercises should be taught sitting up although they can be done lying down. Look directly at the children and have them look directly at you. This is the key to holding their attention!

CHALK CIRCLE

Lie on your back or sit up. Raise your right leg. Pretend that your big right toe is a piece of chalk. Now draw a big chalk circle with your toe. Now draw a little chalk circle with your toe. Go in the other direction, and draw a big circle and a little circle. Now do the same with your left leg and toe.

WIGGLY TOES

Wiggle your feet in your socks, either lying on your back or sitting. Wiggle, wiggle, wiggle. Now wave hello to the ceiling with your foot.

PRUNE FACE

Squeeze eyes, mouth together, corners turned up.

SCRUNCH FACE

Scrunch your eyes and mouth, and make your forehead into many turn-down wrinkles.

SURPRISE EYES

Now open your eyes very, very wide. Now close your eyes and let them rest.

KISS THE AIR

Kiss the air 3 times.

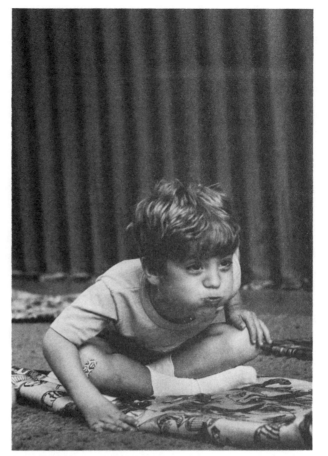

Be a birthday candle.

BIRTHDAY CANDLE

Lift one finger and softly blow out one candle. Now, two birthday candles, blow two candles out; use a little bit more air. Now pretend there are 100 birthday candles; blow them all out! Blow *hard*! Now close your eyes and blow the candles out. Feel the air come out of your mouth.

DISAPPEARING FINGERS

On your mat, either lying on your back or sitting up, stretch arms straight out in front of you and wiggle your fingers. Let your fingers run through the air. Now hide your fingers *very* tight inside your hands so no one can see your fingers. They have disappeared! No one can see them! We may need to call a detective to come and find them! Let your fingers jump out and say, *Surprise!*

Stretch your fingers *very* far apart; hide your fingers again. Repeat the exercise. After stretching the fingers far apart, flap them at the ceiling and say hello to the ceiling, if lying on the mat; if sitting up

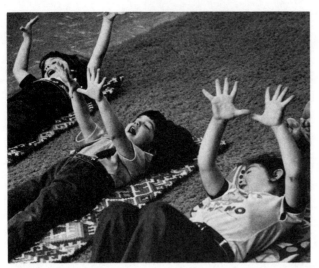
Disappearing Fingers

say hello to someone. Put your hands in your lap. Rest.

PROGRAM 1

Warmup Posture	Part of Body Benefited
Chalk Circle	Ankles
Wiggly Toes	Feet
Prune Face	Face
Scrunch Face	Face
Surprise Eyes	Eyes
Kiss the Air	Mouth
Birthday Candle	Breathing
Disappearing Fingers	Hands
Rock-and-Roll	Spine and Back
Leg Stretch	Legs
Tweak Your Toes	Knees and Toes
Mush, Mush, Mush	Foot
Sleepy-Foot-Baby	Legs and Hips
Neck Roll	Neck
Slide	Spine and Abdomen
Wood Chopper	Abdomen, Back, and Breathing

PROGRAM 2

Warmup Posture	Part of Body Benefited
Heel and Toe Kisses	Calf Muscles and Ankles
Jack in the Box	Spine, Circulation
Feel Your Heart	Heart
Bicycle Ride	Legs and Hips
Sneaky Snake	Spine
Fold Up Your Body and Put It in a Drawer	Resting Pose for Body
Birthday Balloon	Breathing
Quiet Place	Whole Body

PROGRAM 3

Warmup Posture	Part of Body Benefited
Kiss Around the Corner	Mouth
Scarey Lion	Throat
Darling Dolphin	Circulation, Head, Chest
Inch Worm	Hamstring Stretch, Hips
Ice-Cream Cone	Creative Visualization, Body Control
Turtle	Lower-Back Stretch, Legs
Pretzel	Torque Motion for Spine
Bow	Abdomen

ROCK-AND-ROLL

Roll up to sitting position holding onto your knees and roll back being careful to stay on your mat. Keep momentum going forward and back.

LEG STRETCH

Stretch your legs in front of you. Place your hands on your thighs and walk down your legs. Walk over your knee hills; walk down to toe mountains. Then walk back up again. Remember to go over the knee hills.

TWEAK YOUR TOES

Legs are straight out in front of you. Reach down and bring one foot up and rest it on your thigh. Take both hands and tweak your toes, "tweaky, tweaky, tweaky."

Talk to your toes, saying loudly, "tweaky, tweaky, tweaky." Now say "tweaky," softly.

MUSH, MUSH, MUSH

Take your fingers and your thumbs and massage or "mush" the soles of your feet. "Mush, mush,

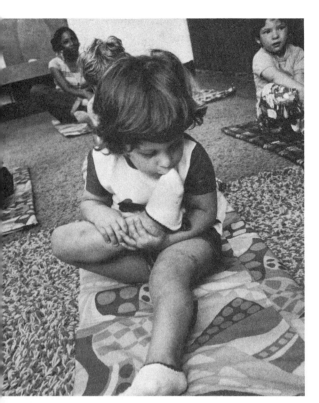
Sleepy Foot Baby

mush." (Say *mush* with the children while doing this massaging motion.) Now "push, push, push." (Say *push* with the children while doing this same "pushing" or massaging motion to the feet.)

Repeat entire procedure on opposite foot.

SLEEPY-FOOT-BABY

Grab your foot with one hand and the knee with the other hand. Now kiss the baby goodnight. Let's sing and rock the baby to sleep, rocking the leg side to side. Now, we'll sing "Rock-a-bye-Baby" and put sleepy foot to bed.

Repeat on opposite side. (One time each leg.)

NECK ROLL

Do slow neck rolls once each direction.

SLIDE (TRIANGLE)

Stand up on your mat with your feet apart. Place your hand on the side of your leg. Let's s—l—i—d—e down your leg. Then, stand straight and s—l—i—d—e once again down your leg. Stand up and repeat twice on opposite leg.

WOOD CHOPPER

Stand with your feet apart. Now we'll cut a great big piece of wood in two. Raise your heavy ax, way above your head. Feel how heavy it is! Take a deep breath; then blow the air all out and bring your ax down hard on the wood. Did it cut it in half? No? Let's try again.

Repeat the exercise, finally cutting the log in two.

Let's go into our Quiet Place by turning off your body factory. Proceed with the relaxation on page 148.

PROGRAM 2 FOR PRESCHOOL CHILDREN (2½–5)

Do any exercise from Program 1, starting with warmups. Add the following postures; do a few or all of the following.

HEEL AND TOE KISSES

Lie on the mat on your back. Stretch both legs up into the air. Let your toes kiss each other. Let your heels kiss each other. Repeat several times, letting toes kiss and heels kiss. Slowly put your legs down and rest.

Can be done lying down or sitting up on mat.

JACK IN THE BOX

Stand up on your mat.

Hold your hands together behind your back for the entire exercise.

Slowly bend forward, lowering your head.

Now, let your Jack in the Box pop up behind you, 1-2-3! (Your arms should be straight, hands still clasped.)

Look at your knees. Hold a few seconds.

Slowly stand up. Inhale and let go of your fingers. Rest.

FEEL YOUR HEART

Stand up and feel your heartbeat. Can you find it? No? Well, let's try to exercise the heart by jogging.

Jog in place on your mat 10 seconds or more.

Now be a basketball and jump up and down 10 seconds or more.

Now let's swim through the air forward, then backward 10 seconds or more.

Stop. Place your hand on your heart. Now can you feel it?

BICYCLE RIDE (A VERY MODIFIED SHOULDERSTAND)

Lie on your mat.

Now roll your hips off the floor; catch your hips with your hands. Let's bicycle up the hill, slowly up the hill 10 seconds or more. Now, let's bicycle faster up the hill 10 seconds or more.

Come down and close your eyes. How does your body feel? Warm? Tingly?

This pose can be modified for very young children just by putting the legs in the air and doing the bicycle. The young child does not need to raise hips off mat.

This is especially good for four-to-five-year-olds.

SNEAKY SNAKE

Lie on your stomach, face close to mat and hands close to face.

Straighten your arms.

Everyone knows that Sneaky the snake has no feet; so let's go back and check out his tail. Look over one shoulder, then the other shoulder. Now look straight ahead and let's rattle the tail. Move feet up and down with a gentle kicking motion.

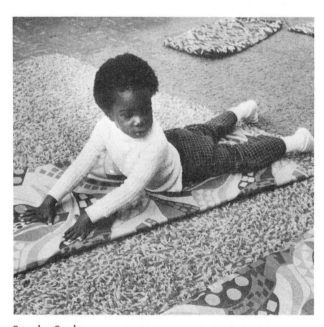

Sneaky Snake

FOLD UP YOUR BODY AND PUT IT IN A DRAWER (THE FOLDED LEAF, OR POSE OF A CHILD)

Onto your knees and make your body really, really small, so you can put it away in a drawer.

Bring your head close to your knees, your chest close to your thighs, and arms close to your body.

BIRTHDAY BALLOON

Now we'll blow your birthday balloon way up.

Place your hands together and arms straight out in front of you.

Inhale and spread your arms way apart, making the balloon very large. What happens to a balloon when it grows too large? It goes *pop*! Bring your hands together. Exhale and *pop*. (Clap hands together!)

Repeat. Do 3 times.

QUIET PLACE

Now go into your Quiet Place, turning off your body factory.

PROGRAM 3 FOR PRESCHOOL CHILDREN (2½–5)

Do any warmups from Programs 1 and 2; don't omit breathing. Add on your child's favorite from 1 and 2; then one new pose from 3. Your program should last about 15 minutes, always ending with Quiet Place.

KISS AROUND THE CORNER

First, kiss the air. Then try and kiss around a corner one way, then another.

SCAREY LION

Sit on your knees. Place your hands on your knees.

Open your Surprise Eyes very wide.

Open your mouth very wide and stick your tongue way out.

Now give a quiet roar in my direction, not too

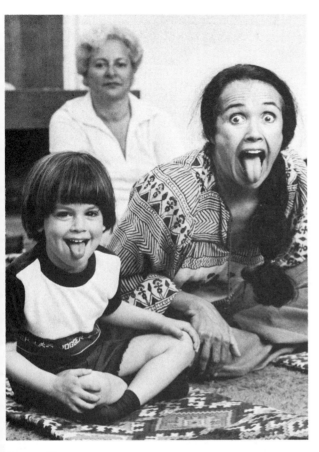

Scarey Lion

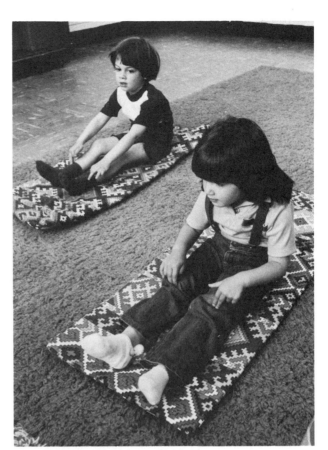

Inch Worm

loud. You do not want to hurt your throat, but be a scarey lion! Let's roar at the assistant in the room. Now a quiet roar at your friends on either side of you.

    Close your eyes and feel your face and tongue.
    Do 3 times.

DARLING DOLPHIN (MODIFIED INVERTED POSE)

    Sit on your knees.
    Make a nest with your hands. Put your elbows on the floor.
    Bring your head down close to your hands and raise your seat (bottom) up toward the ceiling.
    Now pretend you are diving into the water.
    Look at the ceiling with your eyes.
    Hold 5 seconds and come out of the water.

INCH WORM (STANDING FORWARD BEND)

    Sit near the top of your mat.
    Face me and bring both ankles together.

    Place both hands on thighs. Slowly walk your fingers down your legs.
    Bend your knees, placing fingers on the floor. Now, walk your fingers around your back, 6 inches out in front of you. "Walk walk, walk."
    Then inch your feet up to your fingers just like an inch worm moves. Walk your fingers out in front of you once again and inch your feet up to fingers.
    Then go back backward and walk fingers back up ankles, over the bumpy knees, up thighs to hips.

ICE CREAM CONE

    Stand on your mat.
    Bring your hands together, up over your head. Stretch!
    Think of yourself as your favorite ice cream cone. What flavor are you? What color are you?
    You are so yummy; pretend that someone begins to eat you slowly.
    You are so good to be eaten very, very slowly!
    Feel yourself becoming smaller and smaller. Feel yourself melting until there is nothing left to eat. Very slowly, ease the body down to the mat simulating a melting, well-munched-on ice cream cone.
    Now sit up.

Hatha Yoga Exercises for Preschool Children

TURTLE

Sit on your mat with your legs apart.

Lean forward and place both hands in front of you on the floor.

Now, we are turtles. Let's go into our shells.

Place your hands beneath your bent knees. Slide your hand even farther beneath your knees.

Now we are in our turtle shells.

Slowly pull your hand out from under your knees and sit up.

PRETZEL (TWIST)

Sit on your mat with legs straight out in front of you.

Raise your arms up and play the piano with your fingers. Let your fingers fly up the piano keys; watch your fingers as they fly up.

Then place your hands on the floor close to the top of your right leg.

Look way over your shoulder, keeping your fingers to the floor.

Hold 2 seconds; then raise your hands and watch your fingers fly down the piano keys.

Repeat the Pretzel on opposite side of the body.

Repeat Birthday Breathing from Program 2.

BOW

Lie on your mat on your stomach.

Bend your knees. Reach back and grab your ankles.

Lift your knees off the floor. Now lift your chest off the floor. Look up toward the ceiling.

Don't hold your breath. Remember to breathe as you lift your chest off the floor.

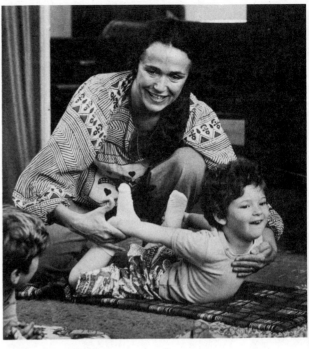

Bow

Let go of your ankles and relax your whole body, just as if you are a lump of butter on top of pancakes. Melt into your mat just like that lump of butter. Then take a deep breath. Slowly release the air and melt once again.

ROCKING BOW

Repeat the above, but this time rock forward and back, forward and back.

Now, you have three healthy, safe, easy programs to follow. Vary these suggestions in any way that you wish. Most of all, make it fun for the kids, and you will have a wonderful time, too!

Yoga has become an important part of the actor's training at the American Conservatory Theater in San Francisco (ACT). ACT offers a three-year training program and is accredited to give a Master of Fine Arts in Acting. Hatha Yoga is included in both programs. ACT is the largest resident professional company in the U.S., with some 75 students in residence and more than 500 short-term trainees. It is unique in that its public performances are concurrent with, and inseparable from, a continuing program in theater training. At ACT opportunities for creative growth have the highest priority.

It is here that Bonita Bradley has been teaching Hatha Yoga since 1970. A professional actress who has also studied Yoga in India, she has developed a special Yoga Program for Performing Artists.

19
Hatha Yoga and the Performing Arts

Interview with an Actress

Lilias: Tell me about the founder of ACT, Bill Ball. It must have been quite unusual to have Yoga as part of theater studies 10 years ago.

Bonita: Yes, it was. ACT has always sought to complement the traditional with new and experimental training methods, exploring the use of disciplines formerly not associated with the performing arts, such as Yoga, and the Alexander Technique of body alignment.

Bill Ball has a very positive outlook on life and works constantly on his own creative, mental, and spiritual development. He encourages fellow actors and students to do the same. One of his primary goals has been to bring each actor-student closer to the fulfillment of his or her own potential, thus helping to raise the standards of American acting as a whole. He practices Yoga and meditation, and he has designated a room at ACT for meditation with a sign over the door so it is used only for that purpose. The rest of the building might be noisy and crowded, but there students can go and center themselves through meditation.

Lilias: The term *spiritual* is often used in Yoga, but when it's used in the living theater, what does it mean?

Bonita: I use the term *spiritual* not in a religious sense, but rather to describe what happens between actor and spectator. It is the potential of the living theater to celebrate and extend the human experience. Isn't this what Yoga is all about?

In the theater we talk a lot about being centered. One of the first things I noticed was that the very good actor is in touch with an internal energy, an energy of the universe, if you will, and projects this out into the audience. Yoga is one of the ways to get in touch with, and bring out, this energy within.

Lilias: Can you give me an example?

Bonita: I see my students constantly trying to free the self from their physical and emotional tensions that act as blocks and hold back that flow. This freeing-up process often comes through physical movements and workouts. Then, Hatha Yoga begins when you face yourself, challenging yourself to break through your own limitations. Yoga brings new awareness and freedom to all levels of one's being. What actually seems like new physical breakthroughs, such as releasing a tight shoulder or the chest, also has far-reaching psychological effects. In acting, as in life, you are working to discover your whole being, the real transformation and freedom being new flexibility on all levels.

Lilias: Practically speaking, does Yoga help with stage fright or nerves?

Bonita: Acting is a highly pressured business. Yoga is the perfect and natural way to calm frayed nerves, renew energy and inspiration. Certain poses help to calm the nervous system or revitalize the tired actor. Increased confidence helps to overcome stage fright. Yoga does give confidence!

Lilias: I know my own studies of Hatha Yoga have made me much more conscious not only of

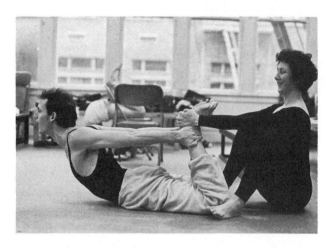

"Various movements work on opening the chest, and so change the quality and depth of voice." Bonita Bradley.

the front of my body, but also of the back of the body.

Bonita: Yes, and you can imagine how very important body alignment is on stage! Here every idiosyncrasy is magnified! Body alignment becomes terribly important. Also, physically standing on the stage can be difficult. The stage we work on is on a slant. This creates lower-back strain and can be released with postures for the lower back and shoulders.

Another area where Yoga helps is with voice work. Various movements depend on opening the chest, and so change the quality and depth of voice, and relax the voice. The actor and the singer need to relax the tightness by opening up the muscles of the chest. Opening the chest is important and helps you keep the voice in good shape. It also expands the lung capacity. Two exercises for doing this are Hanging over the Bed Backwards and The Bridge.

Lilias: What is the most important benefit the actor can have through Yoga?

Bonita: I would say maybe the lesson of being fully aware of the moment, to be here now. Good acting requires intense concentration and awareness of what one is doing on stage. This singleminded attention is also needed during the execution of postures. The ability to be inside the character at every moment distinguishes a really good actor from an average one.

Interview with an Opera Singer

Noel Tyl, dramatic baritone, a specialist in Wagner, national leader in astrology and author of 16 best-selling textbooks on the subject, is truly a giant of a man. He is blessed with a magnificent voice, fine health, and a weight of 262 pounds, which is perfect for his 6'10" frame.

There can be incredible physical and mental demands made upon the luminaries of the opera world. To this Noel Tyl is no stranger. In the role of Wotan, Noel carries a 15-foot spear, which he gingerly throws, often from one hand to another, as he performs for two continuous hours on a slanted stage, wearing a 20-pound costume.

Bones, muscle texture, and body configuration affect a singer's voice. Good health is important, too. With busy schedules, constant travel, long rehearsals in dusty halls, how does one cope and maintain good health?

We sat in his dressing room and had fun talking and stretching.

All of us complain about not getting enough exercise! It's very hard for us to find the right sort of exercise program. It is dangerous for a singer to jog. You're taking in all sorts of air, polluted and cold in the winter. You're also using the wrong breathing mechanism when you run. Just listen to a professional boxer. His voice is often gnarled, diffused, and unhealthy sounding so far as vocal resonance is concerned. This type of forced

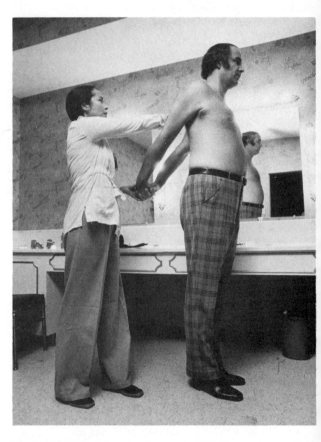

Noel Tyl. "Picture me minutes before I go on standing in the darkened wings with full makeup and costume doing a chest expander."

Lilias, Yoga, and Your Life

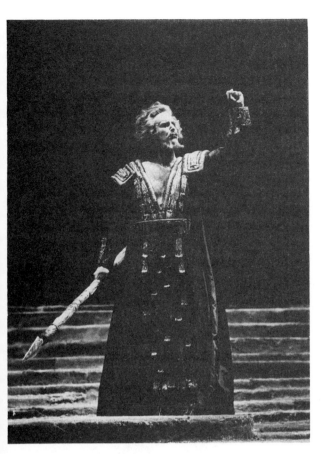

Noel Tyl Dressed as Wagner's Wotan

panting, done for long periods, often can dislodge the larynx.

Swimming is also not too good for the singer. Water gets into the sinuses. There's always a chance of drafts, a chance of colds. Most singers I know do a very careful combination of calisthenics and stretching, sometimes a modified system of running in place to get the respiratory system up.

Exercises seem to have to be gentle. I do some swimming and some simple Yoga for spinal alignment and to bring circulation to the chest and neck areas, and for releasing tension and relaxation. A few singers lift weights and work out in a gym. They are muscular singers, and their sounds are muscular too. They sometimes run into problems when they put too much force into the voice, and the sound wobbles. This is because you have several sets of muscles competing with one another.

You have to work against many unavoidable obstacles in the theater: dusty scenery and stages that make the throat dry out; sitting 45 minutes while being made up, totally immobile and silent; then, like a racehorse in the Kentucky Derby, you are off and running for 2 hours or more. That's extremely difficult. When this happens, you can picture me standing in the wings with full make-up and costume. I do a slow Chest Expander, taking a deep breath, and then go into the Standing Forward Bend. I can feel the release of nervous tension. Months of rehearsals are behind me. The music swells. The curtain opens, and I am truly ready!

CHEST EXPANDER

If you are the kind of person who might need an extra pop of energy during your day, try the Chest Expander. You do not have to be an experienced Yoga student to enjoy the immediate release of tension and the delicious feeling of stretch and energy this posture will give you.

Step 1 of the Chest Expander can be done as part of your personal routine or during an isolated part of your day. When any hectic activity takes your energy, this posture comes as close to giving instant energy as any I know!

Step 1

This phase is easy to do totally clothed; just loosen whatever you have around your neck. Stand with your feet together; tighten your kneecaps; contract your buttocks muscles (imagine you are press-

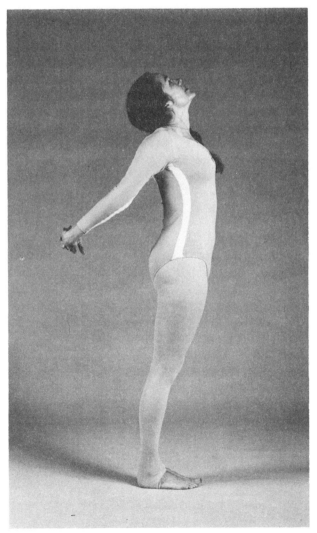

Chest Expander

ing your lower back to a wall); interlock your fingers behind your back; and then rotate your shoulders.

Straighten your elbows. Inhaling, pull shoulders down from your ears.

Exhale and smoothly raise your arms, keeping your elbows straight.

Inhale and lift your chin toward the ceiling. Feel that you are lifting up your breastbone and that your ribs are separating. Hold your breath in this position for three seconds without leaning forward; stretch upward. Then, exhale and let your arms hang loosely at your side. Close your eyes and observe the warmth and lightness of your shoulders, chest, and arms. Imagine tension and fatigue draining down and out the center of your hands. Repeat.

Step 2

Follow the above directions (Step 1).

Firmly holding onto your hands, inhale and lift your chin toward the ceiling. Then, exhaling, stretch your upper body forward, bending slowly at the waist and leading with your chin. Do not let go of the slight pressure in the upper curve of your neck as you stretch forward. When you can go no farther forward, tuck in your chin, nose, and forehead toward your knee, bringing your arms up and over your head.

Do not force or bounce as you hold this Forward Bend pose. Squeeze your shoulder blades together gently. Pull your shoulders down from your ears. Hold this Forward Bend position 5 seconds or longer. Inhale and lengthen and elongate your abdominal muscles. Exhale as your chest comes closer to your thighs.

Step 3

Inhaling, raise your forehead, nose, and chin, stretching your chin toward the wall in front of you; then elongate and straighten your spine. Exhaling, return to standing straight position. Repeat Chest Expander, Steps 1, 2 and 3.

Variation

Go through Steps 1 and 2. While bending forward raise your arms as high as possible; then slowly and gently sway your arms to the right by letting your right hand pull the left hand. Repeat on opposite side. Keep your shoulders steady and quiet throughout the movement. Proceed to Step 3.

In Step 1, clasp your hands together, straighten your elbows, and then turn your hands inside out. Palms down to floor.

Helpful Hints

Whenever you are in this type of standing-forward bend, check to be sure your upper-body

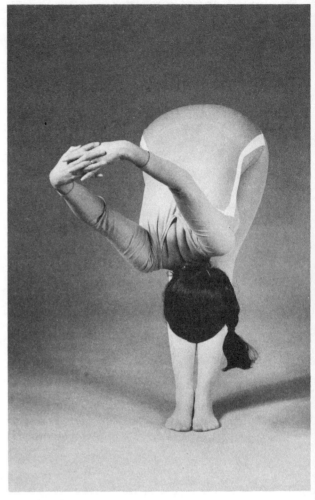

Chest Expander, Variation

weight is on the balls and toes of the feet as well as the heels. Too much weight distribution on the heels can cause a back knee or hyperextension of the back of the knees. This condition is to be avoided.

Hands wet from perspiration will slip easily from their locked position during the intense arm stretch.

I suggest that to maintain this lock firmly, press the pads of your fingers into the hollow of the opposite knuckle.

HATHA YOGA PROGRAM FOR THE PERFORMING ARTS

This is an especially designed beginner program for men and women in the performing arts. Special attention is given to the shoulders, lungs, and pelvis, which are stretched and moved, thus increasing their strength, flexibility and blood circulation. Many of the exercises in the first week, such as Push Away and Hulk are from *All Shoulder Work*, designed to strengthen and increase flexibility in the shoulder area, page 28.

The pelvic girdle (lower-back and abdominal area) will be strengthened by *all* starred exercises of the second and third week. These exercises come from "Back Talk," chapter 13.

Fish, Half-Candle, Forward Bend, and Twist also aid in increasing the blood circulation within the pelvis and chest. They are also excellent for spinal flexibility and the nervous system.

The emotional-stability routine, pages 84–85, chapter 12, is fantastic for release of nervous tension! You also might be very interested in the creative visualization exercises from this chapter.

Relaxation is the frosting on the cake. It promotes a better night's sleep, and increases your confidence in your ability to relax during the day or in any stressful situation.

First Week

All tension relievers
Neck Tilt
Shoulder Roll
Neck Roll
Rag Doll
Chest Expander
Fish Over a Barrel
Push Away
Rope Reach
Chicken Wings
Hulk
Over-the-Head Arm Clasp
Breathing and 5-minute Relaxation

Second Week

Repeat all stars from first week, adding
Easy Rock-and-Roll
Pelvic Tilt
Table
Cat Arch
Torso Twist

Dog Wag
Mecca Pose
Complete Breath and 5-minute Relaxation

Third Week

Repeat Chest Expander from first week
Swan Dive
Leg Lift
Swim
Sitback
Arm and Leg Lift
Arm and Leg Lift 2
Complete Breath and 5-minute Relaxation

Fourth Week

Work on Fish Over a Barrel
Half Candle
Beginner Fish
One-Leg Forward Bend with Towel
Easy Twist
Complete Breath using folded sock between shoulder
    blades
5-minute Relaxation

Fifth Week

Repeat the back strengtheners from second and third
    weeks that feel good to you.
Repeat one from above list you do *not* enjoy doing.
Repeat all stars from fourth week.
Complete Breath and 5-minute Relaxation

Sixth Week

Repeat back strengtheners you enjoy from second
    and third weeks.
Repeat one from the above weeks you do *not* enjoy
    doing.
Repeat all stars from fourth week.
Start Emotional-Stability Routine
Do Sitback with Hollow Lake
Complete Breath and Relaxation

20
Yoga for the Blind

The possibility of teaching Hatha Yoga to the blind sometimes comes as a shock to many people. The Asanas, breathing, and relaxation have benefited countless blind students.

Years of inactivity cause many blind men and women to be very out of shape and overweight. Exercise programs, such as jogging, bicycling, and swimming, by their nature require sighted assistants and special facilities for full participation by a blind person. Hatha Yoga gives a blind student a safe, gentle, yet challenging method of exercise that can eventually be done totally *alone*, thus encouraging independence and confidence, as well as mental and physical health.

As a guest teacher, I have always looked forward to Yoga classes for the blind. It is an extraordinary experience to stand in the doorway and look at all the happy, smiling faces. I watch the helpers lead students to their mats on one side of the room. A big, black guide dog snoozes contentedly next to his charge, occasionally raising his head to check out what's going on. Shoes and canes are left at the door. I feel the anticipation within the room. Soon the room quiets down and the class begins.

Interview with a Volunteer Teacher

Minette Hoffheimer is a volunteer teacher at Clovernook Home and School for the Blind, Cincinnati, Ohio. In Clovernook's William A. Proctor Rehabilitation Center, Pat Kambic, orientation and mobility supervisor, helps Minette with the Yoga program. They have been working together for a few years.

Lilias: What kind of changes do you notice in your students during the weeks of classes?

Pat: When you are working in a rehab center and at Clovernook, it is difficult to say that the positive changes in each person are *totally* due to Yoga. There are other classes, influences, etc. However, the Yoga *has* contributed immensely to the lives of some of the blind students. I have found that endurance can be built up in certain students due to Yoga exercises. Many new students get tired just walking from one end of the building to another. For example, we had a girl who had been relying on using her walker; yet there was very little wrong, except lack of muscle tone. At the end of the Yoga training, she could walk up to six blocks, was not winded, and had gained a lot of balance and body control.

Minette: Some students were unwilling to try any movement new to them, such as the Rock-and-Roll. The idea of rolling backward was very frightening. I heard many excuses as to why they couldn't do it, but after a while, they were willing to give it a try and were enjoying it. They had gained the self-confidence and assurance that they could do something they had never tried before. Once they discovered the postures they could do physically, they also felt their range of motion increased.

Lilias: What other changes have you noticed?

Pat: Rocking is something congenitally blind people are likely to do for a myriad of reasons. Because they've never seen people, they don't know that other people don't rock. With Yoga, they become more *aware* of their bodies. They can *feel* themselves rocking—the shift of balance back and forth—whereas, before, they probably were never aware that their own body was in movement.

Minette: I noticed a change during the deep relaxation. In the beginning weeks, there was a lot of movement and fidgeting. By the end, the students really wanted to control their body movements. They enjoyed how good their bodies felt and looked forward to this quiet time.

Pat: Yes, I remember one woman, a very nervous, anxious person with tons of ability, but she couldn't show it! When I started working with her, I treated her as if she were almost on a mentally retarded level. Because she was so anxious and uptight,

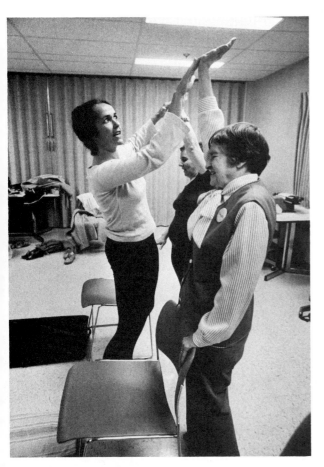

Lilias and Blind Students

she was blocked from doing anything. She *really* picked up on the exercises and relaxation, and soon was doing them on her own! In the end, she took with her what she had learned. She returned home a much more self-confident and relaxed woman. I noticed a big change in her! Even though there were other influencing factors, Yoga definitely contributed to the change.

Minette Hoffheimer offers the following hints for teaching Yoga to the blind.

A class for the blind must be taught by a qualified, experienced Hatha Yoga instructor. Helpers are definitely needed for these classes; these helpers need to be carefully attuned to the class and teacher. There should be one helper per two students, if possible.

The following hints come from several years' experience with many classes. They are listed, not to overwhelm you, but to help strengthen your desire to encourage the practice of Yoga for *all* students, regardless of any disabilities.

Keep the class small.

Warmth and sincerity of your voice are important.

Your students cannot see your smile, but they can hear or feel it in your voice. Good vibes help to cement a loving interaction between teacher and student.

Treat your students like non-handicapped persons. *Don't omit; adapt* when possible. Otherwise, the format should be planned as usual.

It is very important to know the medical background of each handicapped student, particularly with the partially sighted. Inverted postures (Shoulderstand, etc.) may cause increased blood pressure behind the eyes and cause damage. Be aware of what postures should *not* be attempted, and modify others when necessary. For example, a student can place a pillow under the head if lying flat would cause discomfort.

Individual mats are suggested rather than a carpeted floor. The mat gives students their own, private space; they can feel freer with their movements.

It is a courtesy to orient a blind student to new surroundings, e.g., "There are ten students here. We have rows of mats, and you are on the first one. On the mat to your right is Keith; to his right is Nancy . . . . Behind Keith is Sharon, and to her left . . . ." If the blind student is unfamiliar with other members of the class, verbal identification by each person will help him or her connect the voice to the name. "My name is Keith, and I'm to your right . . . ."

Try to verbalize *exactly* what you want to say when explaining an Asana. A blind person cannot visualize himself in space the same way a sighted

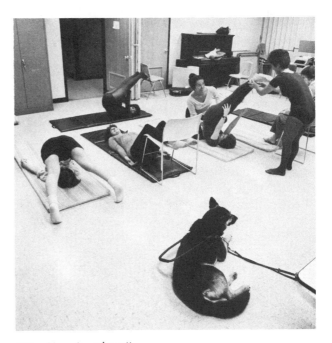

"Don't omit; adapt."

Yoga for the Blind

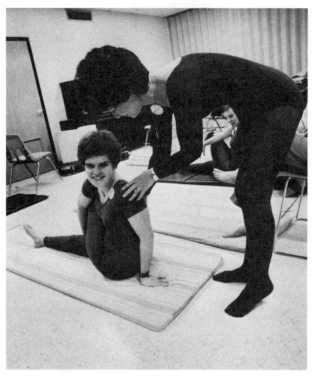

"May I adjust your shoulder?" asks Minette Hoffheimer.

person can. Therefore, use reference points in the room. For example, the concept "up" is different when a person is standing from when he is lying down. If a student is standing, you might say, "Raise your arms toward the front wall and then directly above your head, toward the ceiling." If lying down, "Raise your arms toward the ceiling and then over your head until your arms are on the mat and your fingertips point to the wall behind you."

Don't hesitate to ask your students for feedback. Are your descriptions meaningful to *them*? You can adjust your descriptions to their concepts so that you are talking on the same wavelength.

When I have failed to verbalize a movement properly, I'll touch a student gently, *asking first*, "May I adjust your hip, shoulder? . . ." Otherwise, it can feel almost like an assault. I do explain to the students in earlier sessions that occasionally they will be touched. Now and then, I will ask them if they would like to get a better concept of a body position by touching me. (A hand on my stomach is a helpful aid in explaining certain breathing.) Remember though, the blind can be overtouched. They are being maneuvered constantly through our desire to be of assistance—sometimes to the point of not allowing them enough freedom to develop their own resources.

Use props such as a wall, chair, etc., to help with balance and orientation in space as well as to pro-

vide self-confidence and a feeling of accomplishment.

Utilize other senses. Most students, unless allergic, enjoy a scent such as a light, sandlewood incense. Many enjoy chanting or the sounds of nature like those of the "Environment Sounds" records. When possible, it is pleasant to go outdoors with your class. Make use of all the other senses, e.g., the texture of the grass, scent of clover, call of a bird, a cricket, even negative sounds such as traffic.

It is not necessary to shy away from verbalizing what the students have not seen; just try to equate it with their own experience. In relaxation, you can talk about "drifting on a cloud like a gentle breeze," or "like gently floating in a hammock." Though they may never have seen a cloud, they can imagine the feeling.

Preparing a simple half-hour review for each lesson on a tape-recorded cassette is a valuable tool for reinforcement and practice between classes for the beginning student.

Yoga can be taught to the blind, multihandicapped person, such as one who is partially deaf, epileptic, etc. With some mentally retarded individuals, basic skills and a shorter class time may be necessary. No matter how simple, the exercises can give this person a definite sense of achievement. For the emotionally disturbed, the knowledge that he has the tools within himself to lessen his own anxieties, if only for a moment, is terribly important.

Do not be discouraged if you have people who do not relate to the class. Remind yourself that if you can reach just one person in the class, and give him or her a few tools to use for life, you have accomplished something important.

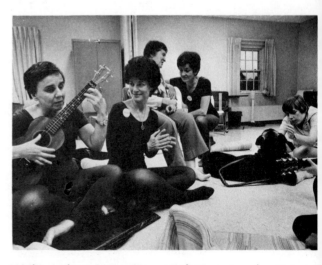

"Utilize other senses. Many students enjoy chanting or environmental sounds."

Lilias, Yoga, and Your Life

Above all, do not be afraid to have a blind student join your sighted class. It will be a positive experience for him, for your other students, and for you. You will be helping to educate the blind student by bringing physical, mental, and spiritual well-being and balance to his or her life. You will also be educating his sighted classmates to realize that this student is just a person like everyone else. Although the person happens to be blind, there is no reason to feel uncomfortable or to act differently.

EXTRA BENEFITS FOR THE BLIND

Because of the slowness of Yoga movements versus fast-paced exercises, the student can become aware of what motion in space is. Yoga makes it easier for the blind student to define motions such as *up, down, fast, slow.*

Yoga helps the blind student understand how the body works. If a blind person has never seen a knee joint in action, he or she has no frame of reference regarding its limitations of movement as compared, for example, to the movement of the elbow. (A straight leg cannot bend forward at the joint. A straight arm cannot bend backward at the joint.) Body language, or the study of body movement, telegraphs to the sighted world personal attitudes. Yoga increases awareness of body.

Balancing postures obviously help because they produce confidence and calmness; students learn they really *can* balance. Balancing also gives the blind student a chance to safely push on the edge of balance and to explore where these edges lie. And it aids the blind person to project a good image.

Yoga brings balance to the right and left sides of the body and helps to offset the imbalance that other forms of physical activity sometimes encourage. For example, working with a guide dog or cane emphasizes the use of one side of the body more than the other.

Being relaxed and more confident makes a big difference in how well and how straight a visually impaired person travels (i.e., mobility). If he or she is very stiff, he or she will walk more slowly, and the more slowly he or she walks, the more he or she will tend to veer.

The more self-confident, calm, and relaxed the blind students can become, the more control they will have over themselves in the midst of anxiety, mobility problems, and stressful situations. Many blind persons are aware of just how tension-producing mobility really is; walking to work, cross-

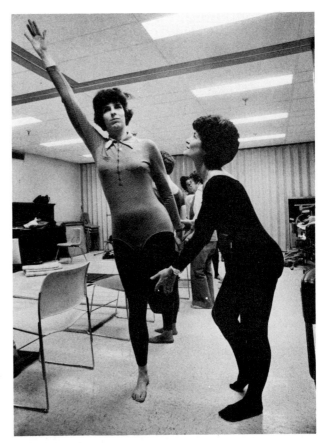

Balance postures give the blind student a chance to explore where the edges of balance lie.

ing the street, riding public transportation. The more one travels, the more tension is produced. Yoga exercises can relieve much of these physical tensions.

By learning to recognize tension, and then by releasing it, the student allows the muscles to work more efficiently and effectively.

The blind are not distracted by visual disturbances and can learn to concentrate and listen to their own mental and physical needs. By learning Yoga concentration and mind techniques, they can use them in other classroom work as well as other daily activities.

The more concepts the blind are given and can practice, the deeper the awareness in *everything* they do.

WHAT YOGA MEANS TO ME

A class at Clovernook was asked to express "what Yoga means to me." These are some excerpts from statements received:

Yoga has helped me in many ways, although it has not come overnight. The first thing I gained was the satisfaction of doing something well, whether it was playing piano in public, body coordination, or learning to relax. It has built up my endurance and resistance against fatigue. Most of all, it has helped me to be considerate of others, to understand their goals and aspirations in life, as well as my own. I now look upon each person as one of life's treasures.

—MARJORIE BOOK, author of *Marjorie's Book;*
Collected Poems of Marjorie Book
Clovernook Press, Cincinnati, Ohio

Yoga is an exciting, ongoing adventure that has radically changed my life. My body awareness has been increased. I am better able to deal with my body's limitations as well as its strong points. Yoga has enabled me to gain greater peace of mind, and daily stress has become more bearable. My nutritional habits have changed—less white sugar, more grains. Musically I have been redirected through Yoga. Chanting gives me vocal expression. I perform publicly on several musical instruments with more ease. Yoga has made me more sensitive to the needs of those around me and has put my life into a more balanced state. I would highly recommend this discipline for everyone.

—JANE McIVER

Yoga has caused me to become more optimistic about things I hear happening in the world, as well as to myself. It has taught me to be more relaxed when I am thinking about something and it has taught me to be more relaxed in my actions. I have learned more about muscles that I knew I had, and I've learned about muscles that I never knew I had! I have learned how to use them.

I believe that Yoga is very good because it makes people become more aware of themselves. It is also good for keeping the body in wonderful condition.

—NANCY McMULLEN

If you are a blind student just beginning your practice of Hatha Yoga, I think using the practice schedule from the Nice and Easy chapter will be an excellent place to start. Also *Lilias, Yoga and You, Book I,* one of the few Yoga books transcribed to braille, can be ordered through the Clovernook School for the Blind, 7000 Hamilton Avenue, Cincinnati, Ohio 45231.

After a few months, you will be more familiar with all the poses. Do find a "real" teacher and join a sighted class. With a little experience and confidence, your schedule will be exactly the same as that of a sighted student.

Working with a partner is very creative and allows both to feel and experience the pose in a little different way. Before working with a partner, close your eyes and sit quietly for a moment. Quiet your inner talking and relax your body. You are about to work as one. Pulling a little too much here or there could cause injury. Your attitude and union of energy with the other person need to be very clearly understood and respected.

Working with a partner is for the teacher or experienced Hatha Yoga student. It is *not* for beginners.

Warm your body well before attempting to work with a partner.

COBRA TWIST*

Warm up well with spinal warmups; then proceed. Your partner is here just to hold your feet evenly to your mat.

Lie on your mat. Feet and ankles together. The partner sits behind you and clasps hold of your ankles.

Place your forehead on the mat to look down your front. Interlace your fingers, cupping the back of your hands.

Inhale; then exhale and tighten your seat, tilt the pelvis and raise your elbows, chin, nose, forehead, chest, and ribs. Inhale and lift higher, squeezing shoulder blades together. Exhale and increase your elongation, working your shoulder blades back.

Inhale; then exhale and twist your body to the right, bringing your right elbow toward the left. Keep working the right elbow back and up high. Right elbow is *not* to touch the mat.

Inhale and come to the center and repeat on the opposite (left) side. Exhale.

Then slowly extend your chin forward and come down. Relax with feet well apart. Take 3 deep breaths.

Variation with a Mat Partner

Do the entire Cobra as directed with hands behind the head variation. It is up to you to communicate to your partner if he or she should change the seated position so you can have more freedom in the position or to lift higher so you can open your chest more. Remember to *tighten* your buttocks muscles throughout the pose.

Come down as slowly as you went into the pose; then switch roles repeating the above procedure.

* Our demonstrator is Mejah Eggerding, teacher and author of *Middle Eastern Dancing*.

21
Yoga with Partners

SEATED COBRA WITH PARTNER

The seated partner plays an important role in this Cobra. The mat partner lies in a basic Cobra pose (page 49), ankles together, forehead on the mat, hands cupped behind the head. The seated partner then stands and places her or his heels on either side of the partner's hips. Toes will be close

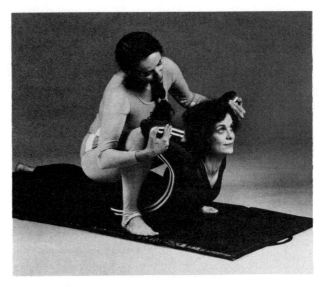

Seated Cobra

to the rib cage. Then the seated partner bends the knees, *leans forward*, and sits lightly on the mat partner's buttocks *behind* the sacrum. The seated partner continues to lean forward and lightly clasps the hands to the mat partner's elbows.

Inhale in unison, slowly pulling your mat partner into Cobra as you guide (not yank) his or her elbows up and outward. Hold. Still leaning forward, ask him or her if he or she would like to go up any higher. If yes, inhale in unison and lift your partner gently up, pressing the partner's elbows slightly out to the sides. Hold a few seconds; then guide him or her down slowly.

Helpful Hints

The seated partner should feel no strain in the lower back at any time. Remember your weight is forward on your feet at all times.

BOW WITH PARTNER

First, warm up well in Bow, page 52.

The mat partner assumes start of the Bow pose. You, the *standing partner*, place your feet on either side of your partner's knees helping to keep the knees 12 inches apart. You then place the heels of your hands on top of your partner's flattened feet. Inhale in unison; then press down on her feet firmly as she lifts her chest off the mat. This press-down motion adds leverage to her posture, enabling her to lift higher.

The mat partner does the Bow as directed on page 52. Hold the pose a little longer, taking advantage of the added leverage as you breathe and lift more into the pose.

LOCUST WITH STANDING PARTNER

Stand and face your mat partner's feet. Your heels are close to her hips and waist. (Adjust your foot position if needed.) Bend your knees, lean forward, and sit lightly on her middle back. Lean forward. Most of your body weight is on your feet, and catch her beneath her thighs above the knees.

Inhale in unison. Exhale in unison on your feet for leverage, and press down, lifting her legs slowly up to the ceiling. Place your elbows to your thighs. Ask if it is too high; adjust accordingly. Hold for three seconds. Your spine is straight, not rounded. Slowly lower her legs to mat. Ask her again if she'd like to go a little bit higher or lower; then repeat the above process.

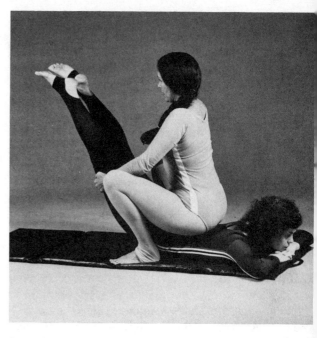

Locust

Mat Partner

Assume Locust Start pose. Ankles together. Place your hands beneath your chin and rest your chin on your hands. Correct your partner's seat position as you must use your buttocks to raise your own legs, and she must not sit so heavily on your back that you cannot breathe comfortably.

FORWARD BEND

Step 1

First warm up well in Forward Bend, page 60.

The *mat partner* assumes Full Forward Bend. You, the *standing* partner, start by sitting on the

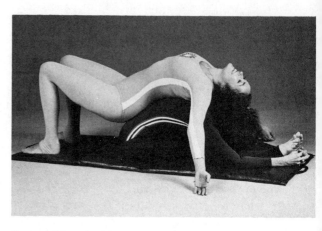

Forward Bend with a Partner (Step 2)

Lilias, Yoga, and Your Life

mat with your back against her back. Your knees are bent; your hands are on your mat. Your weight is on your feet and hands. Arch your spine, placing your spine to hers. Drop your head back and raise your arms from this position. Ask your partner, "Am I too heavy?" (The higher your weight on her back, the more extreme the Forward Bend will be for your partner.) Once she is comfortable, and you have held Step 1 for thirty seconds, proceed with Step 2.

Step 2

Keeping your weight on your hands, lift your seat up a few inches onto her spine, arch back, and mold your entire spine to her back. Then slowly bring your arms out to the side. If this is too much stretch for your partner, lower your seat to the floor. This pose will give you a wonderful stretch across your chest. Breathe deeply in unison as you hold the pose. To come out, release your hands, slide your seat to the mat, taking the weight on your hands.

Step 3

For a deeper stretch for both partners, reach back with your arms and clasp hold of your partner's two big toes. If there is a third person in the room, ask him or her to guide your hands to your partner's toes.

To release, raise your arms, slide slowly down to your mat, and change positions.

SCORPION

First rule in Scorpion is not to attempt it until you are warmed up and totally comfortable doing a Headstand in the middle of the room for 3 minutes. I really find working with a partner in the Scorpion pose a *very* successful way to learn the pose.

Here, Marge and I are working together slowly and step by step on the Scorpion.

Step 1

Place a sturdy twelve-by-twelve-inch (approximate) book against your wall. Kneel down on your mat and place your thumb and four fingers by the corners of the book (note detail). Your lower arms and elbows are in line with the book corners.

Step 2

Kneeling in front of your book, straighten your knees and lift your hips toward the ceiling. *Look at the wall in front of you.* (This feels very awkward at first, but persevere!)

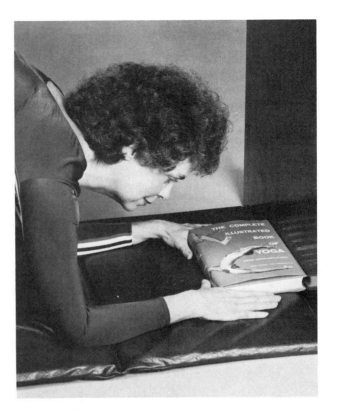

Scorpion (Step 1)

Step 3

Adjust your fingers so you are conscious of having weight on the tip of your fingers. Still keeping your head up, raise your right leg slowly up to your partner's hands. Your partner holds on securely to your ankle. Try to raise your right leg as far up as possible.

Step 4

With your partner firmly holding the right leg as perpendicular as possible, you inhale and raise your left leg slowly up. (Leverage to get you up will come from your held right leg.) Place your left foot on the wall.

Step 5

Your partner then guides your "leverage foot" to the wall. Your partner can then gently hold you around both calves; and the other hand close to your hip for security.

Hold this position ten to fifteen seconds, breathing comfortably.

Stop! Think! Feel! Become accustomed to being upside down. Ask yourself, "Is my head *between* my forearms, *not* my hands? Where are my feet? Am I fearful?" All important questions. Balance comes from correct head position, from the weight to el-

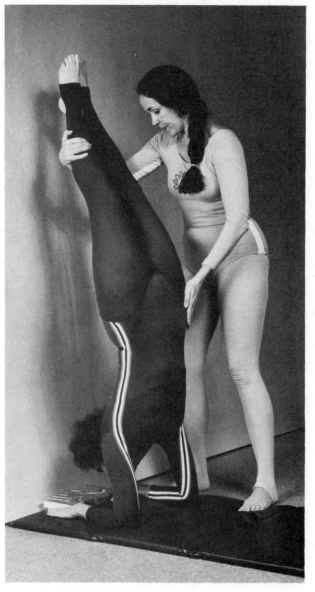

Scorpion (Step 5)

bows and *pads* of tips of your fingers. The body will hold its balance automatically with the correct head-and-arm alignment.

Then come down as you went up, reversing the procedure. Lower the leverage leg last, with support from your partner, so you will come down slowly and in control.

Important: If you find yourself losing your balance or feeling shaky, spring off the wall with your toes, keep your head up, and bend at the waist, bringing your feet to the floor. Collapsing onto your knees or falling on your nose is obviously to be avoided.

Step 6

After a few weeks of going through Steps 1–5, you will feel comfortable enough to start springing away from the wall to find your balance point. Once you are balancing without shaking, try to elongate the spine, tip your pelvis, and extend your heels up toward the ceiling. This takes practice, but it eliminates the lower-back arch, which causes pressure often felt in Scorpion. It is *not* the arch that gives you balance, but the constant lift to maintain the posture—head position, weight on tips of fingers.

As you become familiar, strong, and confident with the mechanics of Scorpion, you will not need a partner.

And if you feel comfortable, strong, and confident in Scorpion, try this posture outside, holding on to the green grass. The leverage you get from the holding of the grass gives you time to work on tilting the pelvis. Should you lose your balance and go over, bring your head between your arms, arch your spine comfortably, and the legs will follow. This is advanced work, so judgment and caution are advised!

Old injuries, recent surgery, and serious diseases of the body can throw out depressing boulders to block your path toward wholeness. Yet you can augment the fantastic healing process of your body (unless there is tear, break, or severe strain) by working gently around the impairment. Studies by the National Aeronautics and Space Administration show that unexercised muscles atrophy quickly. A person can lose one-fifth of his or her maximum muscle strength when immobile for 3 days!

MASTECTOMY

Many women who have had a mastectomy come and study Yoga. Loretta is an inspiration and friend to all in the class. It's been twenty years since her mastectomy. Scar tissue from the treatment left her arm partially immobilized and shoulders frozen with atrophied muscles. She had put on weight due to inactivity, which didn't help matters! Then she and her husband joined my Yoga class.

Yoga has done so much for me! I can now bring both shoulders up under my ears, which I never could do before! I work around my problem when in Dog Stretch or the Plank. With the help of the diet workshop and daily Yoga practice, I've lost 15 pounds and many inches. Life just gets better and better!

MULTIPLE SCLEROSIS

For some time now the Central Florida Chapter of the Multiple Sclerosis Society has been holding weekly Hatha Yoga classes. They are supervised by a practicing nurse, who is also an experienced practitioner of Hatha Yoga. She is assisted by a local Yoga teacher.

Their students vary; some being mobile; some ambulatory; and some confined to wheelchairs. When asked to keep a journal of their first month's Yoga experiences, 87 percent reported positive comments in regard to physical and psychological help.

Some typical responses were: "It is helping my morale tremendously." "I look forward to class." "I feel better after class." In regard to physical changes: "I feel more relaxed." "After the Asanas I was able to walk a few steps without my walker." "Maybe there is hope for regaining my balance." "I was able to do things I didn't think I could do without discomfort." "My blood circulation has so much im-

22
Special Problems

proved. I am now able to wear shoes for the first time in fifteen years!"

Several factors are likely to contribute to the success of such a class.

Yoga's beneficial effects on the mind, the glands, and the nervous system are well known. The group support gives one the incentive to try harder. Yoga is self-reinforcing because of the deep level of rest that can be achieved. Students seem to sense their progress and can expect and see improvements. However, faithful practice was an abolute *must*.

The actual techniques used were the exercises found in any typical Yoga classes. Shoulder and Neck Rolls, Leg Lifts, and deep Complete Breath. Also the classical Asanas were included, such as, Cobra, Locust, and Bow done in their approximate positions. Students were asked to practice each day.

RHEUMATOID ARTHRITIS

Inga Bickford is a brave lady. I want to share her inspiring story with you. Perhaps it will help you or a friend. I know she inspires me!

Lilias: Inga, let me ask you, what kind of arthritis do you have?

Inga: The most crippling, which is rheumatoid.

Lilias: I can't imagine what it's like. How do you feel when you wake up in the morning?

Inga: Stiff and full of pain. I can hardly move.

Lilias: What's it like to brush your teeth?

Inga: Painful. To squeeze the toothpaste, I used to do it with the elbow because I couldn't use my hands at all. I used to just roll myself out of bed.

A few years ago I knew I couldn't go on the way I was. The arthritis was getting worse and worse and worse. The idea of being crippled in a few years and disabled was frightening. I have a restaurant and it's my life's work. I wanted to keep it going. Yet it was so excruciatingly painful for me to go to work every day.

The doctor gave me special exercises, and I've taken special therapy and all that, but it didn't do what Yoga did for me. It was just the gentle stretching and the easy motion like you taught on TV. You would start me just moving my head and just lifting my arm a little. I could not move my arm higher than this. Now I can bring my arms up this high! I can pull my arms all the way back. My doctor is just amazed. I can stretch. I cannot lift my fingers up be-

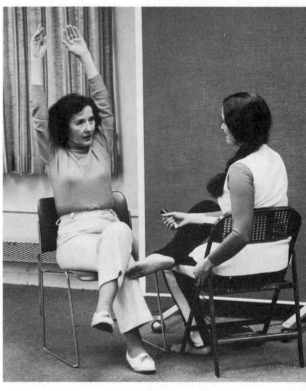

"I know I can handle it, and my outlook on life has changed."

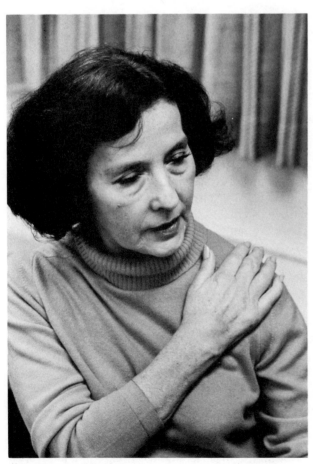

Inga Bikford

cause my wrists are stiff, you know. But look how I can lift my arm.

Lilias: Was it painful at first?

Inga: Sometimes the pain seemed to get worse and worse and worse, and you feel like you don't want to move the joints because it hurts so. Yet when I did move slowly, like Yoga teaches to move, it relieved that pain. The stretching seems to pull my frozen joints apart and brings about circulation. It relieved that pain. I'd be on the floor sometimes crying of pain. I can't do that; I can't do that. Then I get up from the floor after I had one-half hour with you on television, and I'd be amazed. Well, now I cannot live one day without doing my half hour of Hatha Yoga.

Another thing that Yoga has taught me is a positive attitude. I think this is very important, and I want to share this with others, too. The attitude toward the illness that I now have, I didn't have five years ago! I'm not afraid of it anymore. I know I can handle it, and my whole outlook on life changed. It doesn't depress me anymore. And when I have the pain, I know I can relieve it. I have learned how to relax. Nervous tension makes this illness much worse. When I feel tension coming on like in the restaurant when we have people coming out of the woodwork, I feel this tension coming on and my shoulders getting tighter; then I do a few Yoga movements. I drop my shoulders, take a deep breath —all those little things help the pain tremendously. Another sign of the illness is fatigue. Constant fatigue. You get up in the morning and drag yourself to the kitchen and you're tired. It was just awful. Now I'm cheerful again like I used to be and not depressed.

Lilias: Yet your disease is worse?

Inga: My disease is worse. It has progressed in my whole body. I take all the medication that is available. They have tried everything on me. Everything! But my rheumatologist is always so amazed when I start moving around. I can move as well as anybody else. It hurts, but I don't mind it. I'm used to the pain. It isn't as painful as it used to be. I can move. I am restricted in my postures because the cartilage is gone in my wrists, so I do a lot of postures on my elbows. I love the Shoulderstand and the Cobra position. I'm working on the Locust. All the ones I don't like need too much use of my hand. Like the Plow. I do it pretty well and the Forward Bend I'm almost down to my knees with my forehead. Would you believe it?

I have my bad days and my good days. But I'm on top of it. My disease is much worse, but I am better! Inga is better *inside*!

YOGA FOR ALCOHOLICS

Care Unit, an intensive Alcoholic Rehabilitation Program headquartered in Newport Beach, California, teaches Yoga stretches, exercises, and stress-management techniques to its patients. Yoga is helping the alcoholic to live a more relaxed and stress-free life.

Early morning depression can be alleviated or eased with the breathing and stretching. Many patients sleep better and feel a new sort of peace with the relaxation techniques. Many will then pursue classes after dismissal from the care program and make it a part of their everyday life.

KNEE AND ELBOW PROBLEMS

The knee is often referred to as the unforgiving joint because an old injury is often reflected long after recovery. Unlike the ankle, which usually recovers from severe injuries without aftereffects, the knee has a long memory. Serious damage can mean long years of bothersome discomfort. If you can't place your knee in certain positions, get a towel, gather up the ends, then take hold of one gathered end in each hand. Slip the gathered end *behind* your knee. You will look like you are holding your knee in a sling. Keep the towel tight behind your knee and place it in the desired position. This procedure creates a space within the knee area and will make bent knee poses easier.

The Hyperextended Knee

The hyperextended knee is a very noticeable and common problem in human anatomy. It is also called back knee or swayback knee. It is an irregularity in leg structure. The ligaments and muscles over the front and the back of the knee have been permanently hyperextended, and the kneecap has been pulled back beyond normal leg alignment. When seen from a side view, the leg looks like a semicircle.

It indicates knee weakness and *not* flexibility. It also means that a student stands with most of the weight on the heel rather than the ball of the foot. If you have this problem, or a potential back-knee problem, pay special attention to my directions throughout the book, which call for kneecaps to be pulled up.

You must be careful *not* to lock or press your knee joint back. Instead, bend your knee slightly, then bring it back to a straight, but *strong* position. *Then*, raise your kneecaps up toward the thighs.

The floor stretches, such as Dancer's Pose, Wall V, or One-Leg Forward Bend, are recommended for stretching your hamstrings without locked knees. The floor will give you the support and remind you not to go beyond your edge.

Standing Forward Bends can aggravate this back-knee condition. Therefore you can place a blanket or edge of your mat beneath your heels to direct more weight to the ball of your feet.

Hyperextended Elbow Joint

The elbow is a compound hinge-joint that involves the meeting of the upper-arm bone with the ulna and radius (the lower-arm bones).

The hyperextended elbow is due to a shortened upper curve (olecranon process) of the arm rather than loose ligaments in the joint. Girls and women are especially prone to this irregularity of arm structure.

As with the hyperextended knee, there is no way

to correct this problem. It can be improved or disguised by not locking the elbow and keeping it rounded and up. For example, when in Dog Stretch, do not lock your elbows; bend them slightly; then draw them in to a *strong* straight line avoiding a fully extended arm.

THE PRISON ASHRAM PROJECT

Yoga Materials and Prisoners

To request materials or to become a prison pen pal, or to make a tax-deductible donation, write to the main office: Bo Lozoff, Director, Route #1, Box 201–N, Durham, North Carolina 27705.

To donate new or used spiritual books for prisoners, send them to any of the three book projects:

PRISON LIBRARY PROJECT
Box 612
San Rafael, CA 94902

PRISON LIBRARY PROJECT
Box 315
Collinsville, Ill. 62234

PRISON BOOK PROJECT
Box 746
Newport, R. I. 02840

Bibliography

FOR STUDENTS OF HATHA YOGA

ALEXANDROU, EVANGELOS. *Christian Yoga and You.* San Jose, CA: Christananda Publishing Co., 1975.

BALLENTINE, R. M.D., ed. *Science of Breath.* IL: Himalayan International Institute of Yoga Science and Philosophy of the United States, 1976.

CHANG, STEPHEN T. with RICK MILLER. *The Book of Internal Exercises.* San Francisco, CA: Strawberry Hill Press, 1978.

ESSER, HELEN M. *Flexibility and Health Through Yoga.* Dubuque, IA: Kendall/Hunt Publishing Co., 1978. (Can be obtained in bookshops or by writing to P.O. Box 3023, Bridgeton, MO.)

FOLAN, LILIAS M. *Lilias, Yoga and You.* Cincinnati, OH: WCET-TV, 1972.

———. *Stepping Stones to Well-Being.* Three 90-minute audio cassette tapes describing basic Hatha Yoga postures and philosophy. Write to Lilias, WCET, 1223 Central Parkway, Cincinnati, Ohio 45214.

FRENKEL, SITA. *Hatha-Yoga Basic Principles and Practices of Physical and Mental Health.* Washington, D.C.: Today Publications, 1973.

IYENGAR, B.K.S. *Light on Yoga.* New York: Schocken Books, 1966.

JOY, W. BRUGH. *Joy's Way. A Map for the Transformational Journey.* Los Angeles, CA: J. P. Tracher, Inc., 1979.

LEBOYER, FREDERICK. *Birth Without Violence.* New York: Alfred A. Knopf, 1976.

LUBY, SUE. *Hatha Yoga for Total Health.* Englewood Cliffs, NJ: Prentice-Hall, Inc., 1977.

ZEBROFF, KAREEN. *Yoga and Nutrition.* Vancouver, BC (Canada): Fforbez Enterprises Ltd., 1972.

FOR TEACHERS OF HATHA YOGA

BALLENTINE, R. M.D., ed. *Science of Breath.* IL: Himalayan International Institute of Yoga Science and Philosophy of the United States, 1976.

CHANG, STEPHEN T. WITH RICK MILLER. *The Book of Internal Exercises.* San Francisco, CA: Strawberry Hill Press, 1978.

ESSER, HELEN M. *Flexibility and Health Through Yoga.* Dubuque, IA: Kendall/Hunt Publishing Company, 1978. (Can be obtained in bookshops or by writing to P.O. Box 3032, Bridgeton, MO).

FRENKEL, SITA. *Hatha-Yoga Basic Principles and Practices of Physical and Mental Health.* Washington, DC: Today Publications, 1973.

GELABERT, RAOUL. *Anatomy for the Dancer* as told to William Como. New York: Danad Publishing Co., Inc., 1964.

———. *Anatomy for the Dancer,* vol. 2. New York: Danad Publishing Co., Inc., 1966.

IYENGAR, B.K.S. *Light on Yoga.* New York: Schocken Books, 1966.

JOY, W. BRUGH. *Joy's Way. A Map for the Transformational Journey.* Los Angeles, CA: J. P. Tarcher, Inc., 1979.

KAPIT, WYNN, AND ELSON, LAWRENCE M. *The Anatomy Coloring Book.* New York, San Francisco, London: A Canfield Press/Barnes & Noble Book, Harper & Row, 1977.

KUVALAYANANDA, SWAMI. *Asanas.* Bombay: Popular Press Pvt., Ltd., 1931

LEBOYER, FREDERICK. *Birth Without Violence.* New York: Alfred A. Knopf, 1976.

LUBY, SUE. *Hatha Yoga for Total Health.* Englewood Cliffs, NJ: Prentice-Hall, Inc., 1977.

MAJUMDAR, SACHINDRA JUMAR. *Introduction to Yoga Principles and Practices.* New Hyde Park, NY: University Books, 1964.

ZEBROFF, KAREEN. *Yoga and Nutrition.* Vancouver, BC (Canada): Fforbez Enterprises Ltd., 1972.

FOR MEDITATION

ABHISHIKTANANDA, HENRI LE SAUX, O.S.B. *Prayer.* Philadelphia: Westminster Press, 1967.

BLY, ROBERT. *The Kabir Book*. Boston: Beacon Press, 1971.

———. *Gifts of the Lotus*. A Book of Daily Meditations. Wheaton, IL: Theosophical Publishing House, 1974.

COLLINS, MABEL. *Light on the Path Through the Gates of Gold*. Pasadena, CA: Theosophical University Press, 1976.

DE PURUCKER, G. *Golden Precepts*. A Quest miniature. Point Loma Publications, Inc. and Wheaton, IL: Theosophical Publishing House, 1931 and 1977.

GOURE, JIM. *Effective Prayer*. Black Mountain, NC: United Research, Inc., 1976.

LAZARIS. *Lazaris: A Spark of Love*. Fairfax, CA: Synergy Foundation, 1978.

The Narada Sutras, translated by Hari Prasad Shastri. London: Shanti Sadan, 1947.

O'CONNOR, ELIZABETH. *Our Many Selves*: A Handbook for Self-Discovery. New York, Hagerstown, San Francisco, London: Harper and Row, 1971.

RUDRANANDA, SWAMI (RUDI). *Spiritual Cannibalism*. New York and London: Links Books, 1973.

SARAYDARIAN, H. *The Science of Becoming Oneself*. Agoura, CA: Aquarian Educational Group, 1969.

The Way of a Pilgrim and *The Pilgrim Continues His Way*, translated from the Russian by R.M. French. New York: Seabury Press, 1972.

WERVER, EVA BELL. *The Journey with the Master*. Marina del Rey, CA: DeVorss and Co., 1950.

FOR BREATHING

BALLENTINE, R., M.D., ed. *Science of Breath*. IL: Himalayan International Institute of Yoga Science and Philosophy of U.S.A., 1976.

KEYES, LAUREL E. *Toning*. Marina del Rey, CA: DeVorss and Co., 1973.

FOR BACK TALK

BRAGG, PAUL C., AND BRAGG, PATRICIA. *Fitness Program with Spine Motion*. Burbank, CA: Health Science.

FRIEDMANN, LAWRENCE W., M.D., AND GALTON, LAWRENCE. *Freedom from Backaches*. New York: Simon and Schuster, 1973.

KRAUS, HANS, M.D. *Backache Stress and Tension*. New York: Simon and Schuster, 1965.

FOR YOGA IN SPORTS

COLLETOO, JERRY, *Yoga Conditioning and Football*. Millbrae, CA: Celestial Arts, 1975.

ESSER, HELEN M. *Flexibility and Health Through Yoga*. Dubuque, IA: Kendall/Hunt Publishing Co., 1978. (Can be obtained in bookshops or by writing to P.O. Box 3032, Bridgeton, MO).

JACKSON, IAN. *Yoga and the Athlete*. Mountain View, CA: World Publications, 1975.

LEUCHS, ARNE, AND SKALKA, PATRICIA. *Ski with Yoga*. Matteson, IL: Great Lakes Living Press, 1976.

WEAVER, NELL, AND COUCH, JEAN. *Runner's World Yoga Book*. Mountain View, CA: World Publications, 1979.

"NICE AND EASY"

BRAGG, PAUL C., AND BRAGG, PATRICIA. *Fitness Program with Spine Motion*. Burbank, CA: Health Science.

CHRISTENSON, ALICE, AND RANKIN, DAVID. *Easy Does It Yoga for Older People*. New York: Harper & Row, 1979.

FOR PREGNANCY

LEBOYER, FREDERICK. *Birth Without Violence*. New York: Alfred A. Knopf, 1976.

———. *Inner Beauty, Inner Light*. New York: Alfred A. Knopf, 1978.

FOR PRESCHOOL CHILDREN

BRIDDELL, DON AND MOO. *The Adventure of Yoga*. Dallastown, PA: Wood-Mountain Makings, 1978.

CARR, RACHEL. *Be a Frog, a Bird, or a Tree*. Garden City, NY: Doubleday and Co., 1973.

KENT, HOWARD. *My Fun with Yoga*. London, New York, Sydney, Toronto: Hamlyn Publishing Group, Ltd., 1975.

SCHREIBER, SUZANNE LANDSBAUM. *Yoga for the Fun of It*. Preschool Guide Book for Parents and

Teachers. 1547 Shenandoah Ave., Cincinnati, OH 45239.

FOR THE PERFORMING ARTS

Avital, Samuel. *Le Centre du Silence Mime Workbook.* Venice, CA: Wisdom Garden Books, 1977.

FOR SPECIAL PROBLEMS

Christenson, Alice and Rankin, David. *Easy Does It Yoga for Older People.* New York: Harper & Row, 1979.

Joy, W. Brugh. *Joy's Way. A Map for the Transformational Journey.* Los Angeles, CA: J. P. Tarcher, Inc., 1979.

FOR TENSION

Ballentine, R., M.D., ed. *Science of Breath.* IL: Himalayan International Institute of Yoga Science and Philosophy of the United States, 1976.

Benjamin, Ben E. *Are You Tense?* New York: Pantheon Books, 1978

Geba, Dr. Bruno Hans. *Breathe Away Your Tension.* New York: Random House, 1973.

GENERAL REFERENCE WORKS

Bradley, Bonita. "Commentaries on Teaching the American Conservatory Theater." *Yoga Journal* (March, April 1978). Berkeley, CA.

Dowell, Jeanne. "Care-unit Yoga for Alcoholics." *Yoga Journal* (March, April 1980). Berkeley, CA.

Gelabert, Raoul. *Anatomy for the Dancer as told to William Como.* New York: Danad Publishing Co., Inc.

Gelabert, Raoul. *Anatomy for the Dancer,* vol. 2. New York: Danad Publishing Co., 1966.

Herrick, Joy F., with Nancy Schraffenberger. *Something's Got to Help and Yoga Can.* New York: M. Evans and Co., 1974.

Flick, Jim. Bobby Jones quote in Flick's article, reprinted courtesy of *Gold Digest,* from the June issue 1979. Copyright © 1979, Gold Digest, Inc. U.S.A.

Kane, Jeff. "Yoga and Medicine: A Healing Partnership." *Yoga Journal* (January, February 1980) Berkeley, CA.

Seiler, Gary. "A New Prognosis for M.S." *Yoga Journal* (January, February 1980). Berkeley, CA.